# "Read this book"

"If you have hepatitis C and are considering treatment, read this book. *Free From Hepatitis C* provides all you need to know as you travel the path toward being cured."

**Lorren Sandt**
Executive Director
Caring Ambassadors Program, Inc.

# "An informative resource"

"*Free From Hepatitis C* is an informative resource written from the unique perspective of a nurse who is both an expert in the field and a hepatitis C patient who has suffered with the illness. This book is a must-read for people living with hepatitis C, their loved ones, and their healthcare practitioners—especially now that treatments have become much more successful and new therapies are on the horizon. I will proudly display Ms. Porter's book in the reception area of my practice, which is devoted to hepatitis C."

**Melissa Palmer, MD**
Clinical Professor of Medicine
Director of Hepatology, NYU Hepatology Associates Plainview

# "Clear and concise"

"This book is a clear and concise guide to hepatitis C written by an expert nurse educator. Whether you are an individual with hepatitis C, a family member or friend of a hep C patient, or just want to learn more about the most common bloodborne illness in the United States, you will find this readable text an essential part of navigating the confusing labyrinth that is hepatitis C diagnosis and treatment. It's a must-read."

**Diana Sylvestre, MD**
Assistant Professor of Medicine at UCSF
Director of O.A.S.I.S.

# *Free From*
# HEPATITIS C

## YOUR COMPLETE GUIDE
## TO HEALING HEPATITIS C

# LUCINDA K. PORTER, RN

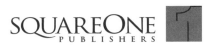

SQUAREONE
PUBLISHERS

COVER DESIGNER: Jeannie Tudor
EDITOR: Michael Weatherhead
TYPESETTER: Theresa E. Wiscovitch
PHOTO: Alicia Berardi of Ivy Photography

The purpose of this book is to educate. It is sold with the understanding that neither the publisher nor the author has any liability for any injury caused or alleged to be caused directly or indirectly by the information contained in this book. While every effort has been made to ensure its accuracy, the book's contents should not be construed as medical advice. To obtain medical advice on your individual health needs, please consult a qualified health care practitioner.

A portion of the proceeds of this book will be donated to support efforts to raise hepatitis C awareness.

**Square One Publishers**
115 Herricks Road
Garden City Park, NY 11040
(516) 535-2010 • (877) 900-BOOK
www.squareonepublishers.com

**Library of Congress Cataloging-in-Publication Data**
Porter, Lucinda K.
  Free from hepatitis C : your complete guide to healing hepatitis C / Lucinda K. Porter.
     p. cm.
  ISBN 978-0-7570-0339-4
  1. Hepatitis C. 2. Hepatitis C—Treatment. I. Title.
  RC848.H425P67 2011
  616.3'623—dc23
                          2011037560

Printed in the United States of America

10   9   8   7   6   5   4   3   2   1

# CONTENTS

*In memory of Emmet B. Keeffe, Jr., MD,
my mentor and friend; and my mother, who taught
me I could do anything if I put my mind to it.*

# A WORD ABOUT GENDER

In an effort to avoid awkward phrasing within sentences, it is our publishing style to alternate the use of generic male and female pronouns according to chapter. When referring to a "third-person" medical provider or patient, odd-numbered chapters will use male pronouns, while even-numbered chapters will use female pronouns.

# ACKNOWLEDGMENTS

Throughout the process of writing this book, so many people helped and encouraged me that it is truly a challenge to know who to thank first. Since Alan Franciscus so generously gave his time to write such a wonderful foreword, starting with him seems like the right choice. My life changed in a most amazing way when I met Alan, the founder of the Hepatitis C Support Project and its website, *HCV Advocate*. Thank you, Alan, for all you have given to the hepatitis C community, for inspiring me to do more than I knew I could, and for being my friend.

I owe a huge debt to Emmet B. Keeffe, MD, MACP, Professor of Medicine Emeritus and former Chief of Hepatology at Stanford University Medical Center, who died shortly before this book was published. I can't fathom a world without him.

There is a special place in my heart for Ginny Morrow, FNP; Brooke Clark, RN; and the Redwood City Hepatitis C Support Group. Thank you for all you taught me. I miss you terribly.

Thank you, Stephany Evans at FinePrint Literary Management. I can't imagine that there is a more perfect agent in the world. Your diligence led me to Rudy Shur and Square One Publishers.

Rudy, you were consistently gracious with your time and wisdom. Thank you for your calm, sensible encouragement, and for believing in me.

Michael Weatherhead, my editor at Square One Publishers, you are every writer's dream. Not only are you a magician, you are a delight to work with, so thank you.

Deborah Appel, you are my best friend, teacher, and pro bono editor. Who knew that our friendship would have deepened in yet another way? You brought coherence and beauty to this book. I hope you know how indebted I am to you.

Thank you, Karen Ely, Steve Goodman, Theresa Hodges, Robert Kressly, Paul Matlock, and Irene Mann. Your input made this book much better than it would have been otherwise. Thank you, David (C.D. Mazoff, PhD) for feeding me ample doses of humor just when I needed it.

Thank you, *Sierra Writers*, particularly the writers in the critique groups. John Skinner inspired me beyond my natural limits and continues to do so, although he did not live to see this book in print. Thank you, Delynn M.Tjoelker, Bruce Bolinger, Paul August, and Jan Westmore for your constructive feedback. A special thank you goes out to Claudine Chalmers for helping me find the title to this book.

Sherry, I hope you know how much you give me, because there isn't enough space to express the volume of appreciation I have for you. Publication of your book inspired me to complete this one.

Thank you to my mother, father, and stepmother, none of whom ever questioned my need to put words on paper.

Amelia, you put up with me through two treatments and spoke truths to me that I could not see, like a kid who points out that the emperor is naked but still sticks around for the parade.

Finally, thank you, Ed. You shopped, cooked, and loved me through two treatments and the writing of this book. Every woman should be so lucky.

# FOREWORD

"I'm cured!" I never expected to utter those words when I was diagnosed with hepatitis C in 1996. While a diagnosis of HCV is always a life-changing event, at that time, little was known about the chronic virus or how to live with it, and what was known was confusing and contradictory. According to some sources, being infected with HCV was nothing to worry about; according to others, it was fatal. Upon recognizing a need for reliable information, I founded the Hepatitis C Support Project (HCSP). Over the years, the HCSP along with its website, the HCV Advocate, has grown tremendously, becoming one of the most trustworthy organizations in the field. The key to this success has been the participation of Lucinda Porter, whose involvement has helped make the project what it is today. Her experience with the virus comes not only from her work with prominent liver specialists as a clinical trials coordinator at Stanford University Medical Center, the countless academic conferences she has attended on the subject of HCV, the articles she has written for numerous HCV organizations, and the HCV support groups she has facilitated, but also from being an HCV patient herself.

Shortly after starting the HCSP, I met Lucinda at a meeting to organize a hepatitis C conference in California. I felt an immediate kinship with her, due to her knowledge of the disease and commitment to educating and supporting the people affected by it. Not long after our first discussion, I asked Lucinda if she would consider writing for the HCV Advocate newsletter. She accepted, and her column, HealthWise, ran in our second issue, in February 1998. Since that time, Lucinda has continued as a contributor, and her role within the HCSP now includes another monthly column called HCV SnapShots, as well as authorship of hundreds of HCV fact sheets, comprehensive guides, and brochures. Over the years Lucinda and I have collaborated on many projects, including coauthoring articles and publications, and organizing support groups, training workshops, and various seminars. One of our most important collaborations, however, began when we went through treatment at the same time. We helped each other through the experience, sharing advice, support, and encouragement—elements that are crucial to the success of HCV therapy.

If you are reading this book, you are most likely considering treatment. To successfully complete the program, it is wise to take advantage of every available resource, including family, friends, medical providers, support groups, and now, this comprehensive text. *Free from Hepatitis C* provides a wealth of information and advice to help your journey go as smoothly as possible. It details the basics of hepatitis C, such as transmission and prevention, diagnostic tests, and the progression of the disease. It also describes actions you can take to attain and maintain a healthy lifestyle as you prepare for and begin therapy. It explains what to expect during treatment, how to manage the side effects and identify which ones need medical attention, how to find support, and how to handle the subject in your work life and private life. Finally, it discusses what to expect once treatment has ended. And, of course, Lucinda presents all this information in a way that combines her knowledge, personal experience, compassion, and unique sense of humor.

It is truly remarkable that HCV treatment has advanced to the point where the word "cure" can be used to define its response in a majority of patients. Even more encouraging is the fact that many scientists believe that HCV medication will one day be able to cure every single case of the disease. But new and better drugs are only part of the equation. The other critical aspect is the guidance that people receive while on treatment, which this book provides. Lucinda's informative text gives HCV patients the best odds of successfully completing treatment and, hopefully, being cured.

As I mentioned at the outset of this foreword, HCV therapy cured me. I can't even begin to tell you how much better I now feel, both physically and emotionally. I wish that every HCV sufferer could experience the sheer joy of living without the virus. You are about to begin a journey with Lucinda that may bring that wish a little closer to reality.

—ALAN FRANCISCUS
Executive Director, Hepatitis C Support Project
Editor-in-Chief, HCV Advocate,
www.hcvadvocate.org

# INTRODUCTION

*Freedom is nothing but a chance*
*to be better.* —Albert Camus

I n 1988, I was infected with a virus that didn't even have a name,
let alone a treatment. It has since been labeled chronic hepatitis
C virus, or HCV. As a nurse working with HCV patients, for many
years, I had little to offer but hope for better HCV treatment, as
success rates were so low. Now, that hope is a reality. It is true that
HCV therapy does not cure everyone 100 percent of the time, but
the odds of beating the disease are excellent and improving. Those
patients who don't permanently eliminate HCV still reap health
benefits that are usually worth the investment. At this time, I believe
that there is more to lose by not trying treatment than by giving it
a shot.

I know, it's easier said than done. After reading the list of side
effects associated with HCV drugs, my first reaction was that it
would be better to take my chances with the disease rather than
attempt therapy. It did not occur to me that HCV treatment might
not be as bad as I had heard or imagined. Choosing between living
with HCV and going through treatment can seem like being wedged
between a rock and a hard place. But what if the hard place is not
as hard as you think it might be? Or what if it is hard but temporary and quite bearable? I have learned firsthand that ordinary people, despite their fears and reservations, can successfully complete

1

HCV treatment. I have witnessed many patients finish it. Some were so afraid that it took them years to make up their minds before agreeing to the protocol. Their strength inspired me to try HCV therapy for myself; their experiences showed me the easiest way through it; their stories moved me to share this message of hope.

## MY STORY

When I was thirty-five, a blood transfusion both saved and forever altered my life. At the time, medical science was well aware of viruses such as HIV (the virus that causes AIDS), hepatitis A, and hepatitis B, as well as other microorganisms that had previously threatened the safety of transfusions, so the blood supply was thought to be safe. No one knew that there was another virus flourishing in the United States and around the world, and thus, in the blood supply. Two months after my blood transfusion, I felt severely fatigued. Laboratory tests showed liver problems. After a liver biopsy, I was diagnosed with non-A, non-B hepatitis. A year later, science isolated the virus and named it hepatitis C, or HCV. After a while, the exhaustion eased, so I thought my body had recovered from HCV on its own. I had no idea that the illness was taking up permanent residence in my system, multiplying and slowly destroying my liver.

Although the initial relentless fatigue improved, it never completely vanished. I knew the virus hadn't left my body. Tired of being tired all the time, I consulted a liver specialist. It was 1997, and treatment for HCV was relatively new, consisting of a single medication called *interferon alfa*. The probability of responding to the drug was extremely low, but I didn't let the odds stand in my way. I figured that the medication worked for some patients, why couldn't it work for me? For three months, I waded through treatment, stopping after the virus did not budge.

By 2003, HCV treatment consisted of *pegylated interferon* in combination with *ribavirin*. Success rates were much higher, the drugs were easier to tolerate, and the medical community knew significantly more about good side effect management. Therapy was much easier the second time. There were no side effects during the first couple of weeks, and when they showed up, they were gradual and tolerable. My appetite diminished and I lost some weight, which I needed to lose anyway. At times, I was grouchy and depressed. Sometimes my brain felt like gelatin—a condition that patients call "brain fog." (I couldn't find where I parked car a few times, and I ran out of gas once. On another occasion, I couldn't understand why my car keys wouldn't fit into the ignition, only to discover that I was trying to start someone else's car, which wasn't even the same make or color as mine!) Normally active, I spent evenings on the sofa, becoming all too acquainted with television. Occasionally, I had insomnia, but rather than toss and turn, I found comfort in reruns of *I Love Lucy* and *Barney Miller*. Sometimes treatment was so easy, sometimes it was difficult, but it was always tolerable. And after three months, my HCV was undetectable, which encouraged me to stick it out. The laundry got done, the bills paid, and occasional crises were handled. I assure you, I am not superhuman. If I was able to deal with the side effects of HCV treatment and complete therapy, so can you.

## WHAT TO EXPECT FROM THIS BOOK

*Free from Hepatitis C* is designed to give you more than just hope. It presents practical information that will empower you to make solid choices about your health and provides tools that can help you through HCV treatment. Ultimately, it shows you how to build a solid foundation for therapy, which is the key to its success.

Chapter 1 begins by outlining the basics of HCV. It explains how the disease is transmitted and diagnosed, and relates the history of HCV treatment. It describes the disease's symptoms, its effects on the body, and its risk factors. Finally, it discusses how to build a good medical team, as well as how to reduce the chance of spreading the illness to others. Chapter 2 examines HCV treatment in detail, letting you know what to expect, why you should consider undergoing therapy, and the circumstances under which treatment is not recommended. It lists the drugs you might take, their side effects, as well as the odds of beating the virus permanently.

While you weigh the decision to follow HCV treatment, Chapter 3 can help you maximize your physical and psychological well-being, focusing on the main health concerns of an HCV patient. If you choose therapy, Chapter 4 can walk you through how to prepare for and begin the program. It explains how to follow your drug protocol properly, stay organized, and get the most out of your medical appointments. It even gives tips on how best to conduct your own research, for those times when you feel the need to find answers for yourself. Once you are in the thick of HCV treatment, Chapter 5 will teach you how to effectively manage the side effects, while you will find guidance on how to navigate the professional and personal pitfalls of undergoing HCV therapy in Chapter 6.

Although the last dose of medication signals the completion of treatment, it doesn't quite mark the end of your journey. In light of this fact, the book's final chapter covers what to do as you await the results of therapy, such as maintaining your vigilance against HCV transmission and falling back into your normal routine slowly. It also addresses how to deal with the outcome of treatment, whatever that outcome may be. For those who test negative, it offers advice on how to reassure yourself that you *are* actually cured. For those who test positive, it details the other benefits you will have likely gained from therapy. It also lays out your options for the future, including additional treatment with new medication, which continues to improve significantly.

As both patient and nurse, I've observed a great deal about HCV treatment. I pass along these observations to you, in the hope that you might view your journey as more than just treatment—that you see it as an adventure, an opportunity, and a gift. I wrote this book to let you know that hepatitis C is a curable disease, that treatment is manageable, and that you will eventually get your life back. We live in exciting times. With the introduction of new drugs to treat HCV, the door of hope is wide open and a cure is within reach for many HCV patients. If you suffer from this disease, this book can lead you through that door to a life that is free from hepatitis C.

# —1—

# THE BASICS OF HEPATITIS C

*As I see it, every day you do one*
*of two things: build health or produce*
*disease in yourself.* —ADELLE DAVIS

The statistics are sobering. The World Health Organization (WHO) estimates that approximately 3 percent of the world's population is living with chronic hepatitis C virus infection (HCV). The US Centers for Disease Control and Prevention (CDC) reports that 3.2 million Americans have chronic HCV, which accounts for about 2 percent of the population. Many experts believe that the numbers are higher, as these rates are based on surveys that do not include the homeless, people in the military, or inmates of prisons and other institutions where there the incidence of HCV is considerable. And yet it is a disease that is poorly understood.

If you are reading this book, it is likely that you have, suspect you have, or know someone who has hepatitis C. Perhaps you are scared and confused as a result. If any of the previous rings true, then understanding the illness is the best course of action you could possibly take right now. In addition to defining hepatitis C and explaining how the illness is diagnosed, this chapter reveals the symptoms of HCV, its effects, and its possible progression. It also explains the risk factors for infection and transmission, as well as treatment options, and provides information on how to choose the best medical team for your needs.

## WHAT IS HEPATITIS C?

*Hepatitis* literally means inflammation of the liver. Although some forms of hepatitis can by caused by alcohol, drugs, toxins, and autoimmune diseases, hepatitis C is a viral infection. Simply put, a virus is an infectious germ that is able to reproduce itself only in the living cells of organisms, causing illness. During the first six months after infection, the hepatitis virus, which uses liver cells to reproduce, may clear up on its own. But in the majority of people affected, hepatitis C remains indefinitely, causing impaired liver function that can lead to *cirrhosis* (severe scarring of the liver) or even liver cancer *(hepatocellular carcinoma)*. And unlike other types of hepatitis, viral hepatitis is contagious.

Not so long ago, the medical community knew of only two examples of viral hepatitis, *hepatitis A* and *hepatitis B*. At the outset of the 1970s, however, experts realized that a virus other than hepatitis A and hepatitis B was causing the disease. In 1974, this unidentified contagion was labeled *non-A, non-B hepatitis*. By 1989, Michael Houghton and his colleagues finally isolated the virus, naming it the *hepatitis C virus* (HCV). Since then, additional types have also been recognized.

> *You can't get or give HCV from kissing, hugging, sharing eating utensils, or drinking from someone else's glass.*

## HOW DO PEOPLE GET HCV?

Hepatitis C is transmitted primarily through blood-to-blood contact, such as a blood transfusion. In fact, it is the most common blood-borne virus in the United States. Keep in mind, however, that it is not passed casually. Theoretically, if you had an open cut in your mouth and kissed someone with HCV whose mouth was bleeding, you could get the disease. But the chance of this happening is so extremely remote that it isn't worth the worry. Ultimately, the most common ways in which people acquire or have acquired HCV are:

❑ sharing paraphernalia for intravenous drug use (needles, syringes, cookers, cotton, water, and drugs)

❑ transfusion of blood or blood products, or organ transplantation (prior to 1992)

Although these examples present a much lower risk, HCV infection can also be the result of:

❑ long-term kidney dialysis (hemodialysis)

❑ occupational risks, such as needle-stick injuries sustained by nurses

❑ sexual contact (There is a very low risk for long-term, monogamous heterosexual partners, but it increases by types of sexual practices, number of partners, and presence of HIV.)

❑ sharing paraphernalia for non-intravenous drug use (straws, pipes, and drugs)

❑ sharing personal grooming items, such as razors, nail clippers, or toothbrushes

❑ transmission from mothers to infants during pregnancy

❑ unsanitary tattooing, body piercing, or acupuncture practices

## HOW IS HCV DIAGNOSED?

HCV is diagnosed via a blood test, and may be present in your system whether or not you notice any symptoms. You may feel fine only to learn that you have HCV after donating blood or applying for life insurance. Perhaps you've been uncommonly tired and decide to go in for general blood work, which reveals the virus. The sequence of events that lead to the detection of HCV is not important. The final results are what matter. Ultimately, a number of tests will have to be ordered to determine the nature of your particular case of HCV.

If you suspect that you have contracted HCV, an *HCV antibody test* is an inexpensive way to verify past exposure to the virus. A negative result means it is unlikely that you were exposed. But if the exposure was recent, the test may not be valid and will need to be repeated in six months. A positive HCV antibody test means you were exposed, but does not prove that you have HCV. Since a small percentage of people get rid of the virus on their own, further testing is necessary to confirm the presence of the virus, specifically an *HCV viral load*, or *HCV RNA*, test. If this test comes back positive, you definitely have the disease. If it is negative but your antibody test was positive, then you probably got rid of it on your own. In this case, the viral load test should be repeated, using the most sensitive version available. In addition to confirming that you have HCV, a viral load test measures the amount of virus in your blood. The greater the amount of virus, the harder it is to eliminate. The viral load, however, is not an indicator of your overall prognosis. In other words, a high viral load does not mean you are more likely to have symptoms or develop cirrhosis.

The initial diagnosis is just the beginning. A *genotype* test will determine what strain of HCV you have, which will help determine the type of treatment you should receive. There are six genotypes and many subtypes. Most people in the United States (72 percent) have genotype 1a or 1b. Generally, genotype 1 patients have about a 75-percent chance of permanently eliminating HCV with twenty-four to forty-eight weeks of treatment. Genotypes 2 and 3 have about an 80-percent chance and require a shorter period of treatment. The genotype does not tell you anything about your symptoms, or whether or not you are more at risk for liver damage.

To evaluate the health of your liver, a blood test called a liver panel, or *hepatic panel*, may be ordered. This examination is sometimes part of a bigger panel of tests called a *comprehensive metabolic panel*, or *chemistry panel*. These tests look at liver enzymes, electrolytes, and other chemicals in the body to determine liver function. A *complete blood count* (CBC) and blood-clotting tests are also normally ordered. In addition, your medical provider may want to rule out other liver diseases such as hepatitis A and B, autoimmune hepatitis, and hemochromatosis. If your doctor suspects cirrhosis, he may order imaging and *alpha-fetoprotein* (AFP) tests. AFP is a protein found in the blood and is used to screen for certain types of cancer, including liver cancer. It is often elevated in those with HCV without the presence of cancer, so an abnormal test is not always a cause for concern.

A liver biopsy is the most accurate way to tell what is going on with your liver and indicates what stage of HCV you have reached. There are various ways to perform a biopsy, the most common being the extraction of a liver sample via a slim, hollow-core needle. The procedure is performed in an outpatient setting, using a local anesthetic and often mild sedation. Most patients say the procedure is not a big deal, probably since the liver does not have any nerve cells. Some patients, though, experience a brief period of discomfort.

I have had four liver biopsies. The first one was not fun, likely because the doctor who did the procedure was inexperienced, but I didn't feel a thing the other times. Don't be influenced by other people's negative stories. If my first liver biopsy was the only one I ever had, I would assume biopsies are worse than they actually are; but now I don't fear them. Just make sure the person who does the biopsy has done a lot of them. Ask everyone you know if they can recommend an experienced practitioner. If the biopsy is performed in a teaching setting, ask if a resident will be doing the procedure. If so, schedule the procedure after July so you won't be the first person on which the new resident performs the test.

*Lab tests should be evaluated by an expert, but that doesn't mean you shouldn't become familiar with them. The more you know about the tests, the more you can discover about yourself.*

In some circumstances, blood tests are used in addition to or in place of a liver biopsy. These tests are not completely reliable and have not eliminated the need for a biopsy. Your medical provider may suggest that you get a biopsy done first, and then monitor you with blood tests. A lot depends on the stage of your disease, the availability of the test, and your provider's opinion on the reliability of the tests. Finally, an *abdominal ultrasound* may also be ordered. This is a simple, noninvasive scan that looks at the liver and other organs in your abdomen. Although it does not replace the biopsy, it is a useful test. If you have cirrhosis, your medical provider may use an ultrasound, along with an AFP blood test, to monitor you for liver cancer.

You can keep copies of your labs, but do so with one caveat in mind: If you don't know how to interpret them, lab reports can cause needless worry. Labs need to be interpreted by a qualified medical professional. Realize that an abnormal lab does not necessarily indicate an abnormality. Don't draw conclusions on a single lab result; look for trends. Get the facts before you react.

> *The presence of symptoms does not mean that you have advanced HCV. On the other hand, the absence of symptoms does not mean that your liver is fine. Talk to your medical provider about all of your concerns.*

## WHAT ARE THE SYMPTOMS OF HCV?

There are two phases of HCV infection, *acute* and *chronic*. The acute phase happens in the first six months. The CDC reports that approximately 15 to 25 percent of those exposed to HCV will eliminate the virus on their own. If it endures for more than six months, it is a chronic infection. Unfortunately, the majority of HCV cases are chronic. Most people with HCV, however, are often unaware that they have it. Those that do have symptoms during the acute stage may hardly notice them, or may think they are just "coming down with something." I had classic hepatitis symptoms, which is somewhat uncommon. I felt tired, weak, and achy, and had no appetite, which for me is a 911 situation! Severe symptoms, including *jaundice* (yellow eyes and skin) and rash, are unusual but possible during the acute phase.

In its chronic stage, HCV symptoms may be vague and non-specific. Some people don't notice anything and go about their lives feeling perfectly healthy; others experience multiple warning signs, the most common being fatigue. Additional indications of chronic HCV include muscle and joint pain, abdominal discomfort, and depression. Lab tests frequently show elevated *liver enzymes*, which are a measure of liver activity. (Approximately 30 percent of chronic HCV patients have normal liver enzymes.) The most common symptoms of chronic HCV include:

- digestive problems
- fatigue
- general weakness
- headaches
- joint pain

- malaise and depression
- mental fogginess and short-term memory problems
- muscle aches

Certain symptoms that show up late in the course of the disease indicate a potentially more severe problem and need immediate medical attention. They include the following:

❏ accumulation of fluid, usually in the ankles, feet, and legs *(edema)*

❏ bone thinning and fractures

❏ bruising, either easily or excessively

❏ easy or excessive bleeding from poor clotting *(coagulopathy)*

❏ itching with no obvious cause *(pruritus)*

❏ jaundice (yellow eyes and skin)

❏ multiple abnormal lab results, including tests for liver function, complete blood count, and blood clotting

❏ red palms *(palmar erythema)*

❏ red spots on the face and body *(spider nevi)*

❏ severe mental confusion *(hepatic encephalopathy)*

❏ swollen belly from fluid accumulation *(ascites)*

❏ unexplained weight loss

❏ vomiting blood *(variceal hemorrhage)*

People who never experience any symptoms prior to diagnosis are understandably surprised to learn that they have HCV. Even if you're feeling fine, an HCV antibody test can detect the presence of the virus. In this case, more testing is needed, since a positive HCV antibody result is not an absolute diagnosis of HCV. Remember, a small percentage of those exposed to the virus are able to clear it from their bloodstream without any trouble. In the same way that measles antibodies remain in the body even after the illness has run its course, HCV antibodies linger in the bloodstream. Unlike measles, however, the presence of HCV antibodies doesn't make you immune to the disease in the future. If you are told that you have HCV antibodies, a viral load test should be performed to measure the presence of actual HCV in the blood.

I had HCV for nearly ten years before I started to study it seriously. At first, I got scared when I read or spoke to others about the illness. I thought that my eyes appeared yellow and my palms seemed red, and that the two tiny red spots on my nose looked like spider nevi. I never think clearly when I am stressed or tired, but instead of recognizing this fact, I was diagnosing myself with hepatic encephalopathy. When I broke my foot, I was sure it was due to bone thinning and feared I was just a step away from a liver transplant. My liver was fine. The problem was fear.

## HOW DOES HCV AFFECT YOUR BODY?

The main question that newly diagnosed HCV patients have is "How serious is the disease?" The answer is that HCV is serious, but not in every case. HCV may progress from a mild, barely noticeable condition to cirrhosis or liver cancer. Since we can't predict each person's prognosis, it's best to treat HCV as a potential threat to all who have it. When it comes to the health of your liver, it is better to be safe than sorry.

Although HCV can damage a number of organs and tissues, it primarily affects the liver. With hundreds of functions, the liver is the largest internal organ. You can't survive without it. Thankfully, it is so resilient that even if 75 percent of the liver were injured, it would still function. The strength of this organ, however, has one unfortunate downside: The liver generally doesn't complain when something is wrong. A person with considerable liver damage might not know that this organ is in distress. He may feel some discomfort in the upper right part of his abdomen where the liver resides, but the sensation would most likely be from the tissues surrounding the liver than from the liver itself.

To understand how HCV can progressively affect your liver, it helps to learn the four stages of this disease, which include:

❏ **Stage I:** Inflammation with minimal scarring *(fibrosis)*, which is limited to one part of the liver called the *portal tracts*

❏ **Stage II:** More advanced fibrosis, extending outside the portal tracts

❏ **Stage III:** Extensive fibrosis, known as *bridging fibrosis*, forming a bridge between the portal tracts

❏ **Stage IV:** Advanced tissue damage known as cirrhosis, which may be irreversible, especially as it progresses

Although cirrhosis is the last stage, it is not the end of the line. People may live a long time with cirrhosis, some with a surprisingly good quality of life, and others with huge limitations. When a cirrhotic liver is working well, it's known as *compensated cirrhosis*. *Decompensated cirrhosis* means that the liver is so deteriorated that it can't perform essential functions.

Although HCV can result in liver cancer, liver failure, or death, these possibilities do not become reality unless cirrhosis is present. It takes an average of twenty years to progress to this stage, which occurs in the US population at an annual rate of approximately 20 percent. Every year, roughly 6 percent progress to decompensated cirrhosis, 4 percent develop hepatocellular carcinoma, and 4 percent die. Although HCV does not necessarily progress in a straight line, the longer you have HCV, the greater is your chance of cirrhosis. For those people who develop cirrhosis, liver transplantation is sometimes an option, and has helped many people live long, meaningful lives. In fact, HCV is the leading indication for liver transplantation. Unfortunately, there is a shortage of donated livers. Of the patients who need liver transplants, 10 to 20 percent will die waiting for an available organ.

Aside from illnesses of the liver, some HCV patients also experience *extrahepatic manifestations*, which refer to HCV-related health conditions that affect organs other than the liver. A few of these health conditions are skin problems such as lichen planus and porphyria cutanea tarda, thyroid disease, diabetes, an autoimmune disease known as cryoglobulinemia, a form of kidney disease called

# HCV Stats

Although nearly one out of every fifty people living in the United States has been exposed to HCV, the statistical odds of dying from the illness aren't too bad compared to those of heart disease, stroke, or cancer. In the first decade of this millennium, the annual HCV-related death rate ranged from 8,000 to 12,000 patients, which accounts for a small portion of those infected with the illness. These figures, unfortunately, are all going to change for the worse.

Unless patients are treated, there will be a significant increase in HCV-related deaths and complications in the years between 2010 and 2030.[1] This is because the majority of those with HCV, aging Baby Boomers, have had this virus for a long time, and, typically, HCV causes its greatest damage after twenty years. If HCV is left untreated, rates of advanced liver disease will quadruple over the next ten years—from 30,000 to 150,000 cases per year.[2] HCV-related liver cancer will triple from 5,000 to 15,000 cases annually.[3] In short, if HCV-positive Baby Boomers are not treated, the mortality predictions are grim.

> *Although HCV does not necessarily progress in a straight line, the longer you have the disease, the greater the chance that it will lead to cirrhosis. A healthy liver at age fifty does not mean that you won't develop cirrhosis at age sixty-five.*

glomerulonephritis, as well as non-Hodgkin's B-cell lymphoma. Thankfully, these are all uncommon occurrences. (If you are anything like me, though, you may think that you've been afflicted with each of them at different times—that is, until you come to your senses.) In reality, the majority of HCV sufferers die from something completely unrelated to the virus, though this fact seems set to change. (See the inset on page 14.)

Factors that affect prognosis include gender, age, and a few other circumstances. Men have an increased chance of disease progression, and the older a person is when initially infected, the worse the prognosis. Both alcohol use and body fat, particularly in the liver cells, are also negative influences. In addition, HIV, hepatitis B, or the existence of another liver disease can have a harmful impact on outcome. Finally, ethnicity has been associated with higher rates of cirrhosis-related liver cancer, particularly in the African-American and Asian-American communities.

## HOW IS HCV TREATED?

Even if HCV does not pose a serious threat of death, the disease still affects your quality of life considerably, leaving you to ask, "How can I cure this disease?" Thanks to advances in treatment in recent years, this question can be answered.

*Interferon alfa*, which works by boosting the immune system, was approved in the early 1990s as the first treatment for chronic HCV. Patients self-injected the drug three times a week into the layer of fat just under the skin. Its success rate ranged from 10 to 20 percent,[4] and it had a lot of side effects. In 1998, a major shift in treatment took place with the addition of the oral drug *ribavirin*

(Copegus) to interferon. Scientists still aren't quite sure how ribavirin works, but it seems to display a general antiviral effect when added to interferon. The success rate of this combination was significantly better than that of interferon alone (average response rates were between 37 and 43 percent), but side effects also increased dramatically.[5] There was still room for improvement.

> *When I got HCV, the condition didn't even have a name. Now, there is a name and treatment for it. With clinical trials reporting significantly better response rates along with shorter lengths of treatment, freedom from HCV is possible. Talk to your medical provider about the latest treatments.*

HCV treatment took another step forward with the approval of a longer-lasting interferon called *pegylated interferon alfa-2a* (Pegasys), or *peginterferon*, in 2002. Combined with ribavirin, this regimen was easier to tolerate and had greater success rates. On average, a patient could expect a 52-percent permanent response.[6] The odds increased to as much as 82 percent for those patients with genotype 2 or 3.[7] Only those patients with cirrhosis or other factors that made them less responsive to HCV medications fell below this 52-percent success rate, though a lucky few of them were able to beat the virus.

In 2011, HCV genotype 1 treatment took a huge and hopeful leap ahead with the approval of two drugs, *boceprevir* (Victrelis) and *telaprevir* (Incivek). Because they interfere with the virus's ability to thrive, these medications are known as *protease inhibitors*. They are also part of a larger classification of drugs called *direct-acting antiviral agents* (DAAs). Unlike interferon and ribavirin, DAAs target the virus specifically and stop it from reproducing, or *replicating*. When used in combination with interferon and ribavirin, DAAs provide a powerful assault on HCV.

If you have genotype 1, your medical providers will likely prescribe boceprevir or telaprevir. These drugs are used in conjunction with interferon and ribavirin and have been showing remarkable results in clinical trials. According to this data, patients without a history of prior treatment who take telaprevir along with peginterferon and ribavirin eliminate the virus up to 79 percent of the time.[8] Patients with prior treatment experience who undergo the same regimen display response rates of up to 86 percent, with that number rising as high as 95 percent in one subset of patients.[9] Also showing promise, boceprevir has been achieving response rates of approximately 66 percent. Finally, another exciting feature of these new medications is that many patients may have shorter treatment lengths.

## HOW TO CHOOSE YOUR MEDICAL TEAM

Your choice of medical professional depends on where you live and to whom you have access. The primary physician you choose may be a doctor, nurse practitioner, or physician's assistant. If your primary provider feels it is appropriate, he may refer you to a *gastroenterologist*, a specialist in diseases of the digestive system, which includes liver conditions. If you live near a medical center that offers liver transplantation, you may be referred to a *hepatologist*. These are gastroenterologists who specialize in liver diseases. A referral to a hepatologist, however, does not mean that you need a liver transplant.

Your medical team may also include other nurses, medical assistants, lab technicians, and your pharmacist. But remember, you are the leader of your team. If you don't feel comfortable with a team member, feel free to replace him. You also can try to work things out, of course. Sometimes a medical provider is rushed and doesn't make a good first impression. If someone is recommended to me but doesn't thrill me, I will usually give him a second or even third chance. The decision is yours.

You'll know you've found a good fit when you feel that you can tell your medical professional anything and know that you will be respected. It may take a while before you feel comfortable revealing your deepest concerns, but great healing can come as a result. When I started working at Stanford, I met a patient who had seen his doctor for years but never told him his darkest fear. This man assumed he was dying from HCV, and although he took it stride, he worried about his family. Never once did he tell his physician about this fear, because if he had, his physician would have assured him that he was unlikely to die from HCV. The patient was greatly relieved when he got his facts straight. Later the patient underwent HCV therapy and was cured.

Your medical provider is there to help you heal, but he can only be truly effective when you offer him the information he needs in addition to that which he learns from clinical tests. Don't hold back the facts. On the other hand, if you are treated disrespectfully and you don't think the relationship can be salvaged, then you should consider moving on.

> *Make friends with the nurses and clerical staff at your medical office. These are the people who make the appointments. Extra kindness may help you get an earlier appointment when you need it most.*

## HOW CAN YOU REDUCE THE RISK OF TRANSMITTING HCV?

Worrying about infecting others is one of the most distressing issues associated with HCV. I've heard many stories from patients who agonized over possibly infecting others. One HCV-infected man called me because his toddler had sucked on a washcloth while taking a bath—the same washcloth the man had used to stop a bloody nick after shaving. One woman with HCV cut her lip on a soda can and turned her back to her child for a moment, only to find the child drinking from the same can when she turned back around. The fact is that the risk to these children is more theoretical than real, because there is no evidence that HCV survives the intestinal tract. Worry, however, is a natural reaction. In my experience, patients tend to analyze the many hypothetical ways in which they could infect others, torturing themselves with fear. Fear of transmitting HCV only upsets the patient and does nothing to keep others safe. The best way to deal with fear over transmitting the disease to others is to find ways to reduce the risk and then let go of your fear.

By learning basic safety measures, you can significantly reduce the possibility of infecting others. If there is a potential for blood contact, use precautions. In regards to the risk of passing HCV on to others in your household, the chances are extremely low. Still, experts recommend against sharing personal hygiene tools, such as manicure scissors, razors, and toothbrushes. If you live with others, instruct them not to use your personal items. Emphasize to children and adolescents that it is unsafe to share personal hygiene items with friends or family, inside or outside of the home. Wrap used feminine hygiene products in plastic, discard them appropriately, and counsel family members to leave trash alone. Granted, sharing certain personal items such as nail clippers and toothbrushes presents a low risk, but still there is no reason to do so.

If you are bleeding, cover the wound with an adhesive bandage. Clean up blood spills with a rag or paper towel. A mixture of one part household bleach to ten parts water makes an excellent disinfectant. Place the used towel or rag in a plastic bag, discard it with the trash, and wash your hands. If you cut yourself while cooking, discard any food that blood may have touched, and clean up any area where there may have been blood contact. Any residual virus will likely be destroyed by stomach acids.

Sexual transmission is unlikely, but it is critical to understand the risk, even if it is small. Those in lesbian or monogamous heterosexual relationships are at low risk of getting HCV. Men and women who have multiple sexual partners, as well as men who have sex with other men, are at an increased risk of HCV transmission. This is particularly true for those who are HIV-positive or who engage in practices involving blood or tissue damage. If you or your partner has HCV, decisions regarding safe sex practices are up to you both. Sometimes it is a matter of educating yourself, finding out what the risks are, and learning how to have sex safely. Sometimes, however, it can be an emotional issue. I recall one patient whose wife would not let him touch her. She slept on the edge of the bed, fully clothed with socks and gloves. It took years for her to come to believe that she was not risking her health by just sleeping next to her husband, let alone having sex with him.

If you share drugs or drug paraphernalia, the transmission risk is very high. Ideally, it would be wonderful if drug users all kicked the habit, but not everyone makes that choice. From a medical perspective, avoiding drugs is better than trying to use and share them in a safer manner. But if you decide to share drugs or drug paraphernalia, you should learn how to do so in a way that reduces your risk of getting HCV. The Harm Reduction Coalition provides information about safer drug use, and is a good place to start. (See the Resources on page 148.)

Tattoo and piercing salons are more professional these days, but they still pose potential risk because the procedures involve blood contact. If you are going to get a tattoo or piercing, make sure that the needles, ink, and piercing instruments are fresh and disposable. If you have teens, remember to educate them about safe body-art techniques.

> **Although HCV is an infectious disease,
> it is rarely passed among family members.**

If you have a blood test, acupuncture, or any other injection done, be sure that a new needle is used. Healthcare professionals are required to follow procedures that will prevent the spread of microorganisms, but mistakes happen. HCV has been spread during various medical procedures, including kidney dialysis and colonoscopies. A lab technician in my town made national news when it came to light that she had reused needles and syringes during patients' lab tests. Tragically, I was one of her patients. I still wonder if any patients who followed me also became HCV positive because of her criminal act.

Obviously, if you know you have HCV, you should not donate blood. If medical or dental personnel forget to use gloves during routine check-ups, remind them to do so. They don't need to know the reason, but I always tell them, "I have a potentially infectious disease and you should wear gloves." They usually thank me.

## THE BOTTOM LINE

Now that you are familiar with the basics of hepatitis C, I hope that any sense of fear or misunderstanding brought about by the disease has left your mind. If these feelings should ever creep back in your head, simply remember the following points.

❏ Although HCV needs to be taken seriously, the majority of HCV patients will never progress to liver failure, liver cancer, or need a transplant.

❏ Although the majority of those with HCV will not develop cirrhosis, this is not a reason to ignore HCV or not consider treatment. In fact, treatment is the best way to avoid HCV-related complications.

❏ Although HCV does not necessarily progress in a straight line, the longer you have the disease, the greater is your chance of developing cirrhosis.

❏ While HCV progresses slowly in most people, regular medical monitoring is still essential.

❏ The symptoms of end-stage liver disease are not subtle. An occasional bout of itchiness or forgetfulness doesn't mean you have cirrhosis.

❏ Some of the symptoms of liver disease are also the symptoms of other medical problems. For instance, thyroid abnormalities can cause unexplained weight loss, while depression can cause fatigue. Discuss your symptoms with your medical provider.

❏ How you got HCV is no one else's business.

❏ Diagnostic tests give valuable insight into your health, but a lab test should not tell you how to feel. Plenty of people have abnormal labs but still feel good. Plenty of people have normal labs but feel lousy.

❏ Never make a decision based on a single lab test.

❏ Don't let fear of HCV transmission keep you from living normally. Give and get lots of hugs.

Keep in mind that just because HCV needs to be taken seriously does not mean you should constantly worry about it. In fact, worrying doesn't help a bit. Try not to scare yourself with "what-ifs." Such a mindset can be psychologically paralyzing. If you have HCV, the next step on your journey is to decide whether or not treatment is right for you. The next chapter will help you make that important decision.

# — 2 —

# HCV TREATMENT

*You may be disappointed if you fail, but you are doomed if you don't try.* —BEVERLY SILLS

Y ou don't have to live with HCV. It can be cured. This is great news, and yet some patients are reluctant to undergo treatment. If you had HIV, the virus that causes AIDS, and were told you could get rid of it, I am guessing you would jump at the chance. But HCV is different. It does its damage slowly and silently. Although some HCV patients will die a miserable death, many will live their entire lives barely noticing any of the effects of this virus. Furthermore, HCV treatment has side effects and does not have a guaranteed outcome. For these and other reasons, the decision to undergo treatment is complicated. This chapter discusses why HCV treatment is worth serious consideration, what to expect from it, and the circumstances that might prevent you from taking HCV medication.

## IS HEPATITIS C REALLY CURABLE?

HCV can be permanently eliminated, and thus cured. The word "cured," however, is not universally accepted in the medical world when it comes to this disease. Although some experts use the term to describe the eradication of the virus, they are more likely to define it as a "sustained virological response," or SVR, to treatment. To my ear, this technical term lacks the certainty that the word "cure" evokes, but it is the same concept.

According to numerous studies, 95 to 100 percent of the time, the virus does not reappear once a patient experiences an SVR. In a long-term study of 997 SVRs, only eight subjects later retested positive for HCV.[1] Of those eight, only one had completed a full course of treatment, and the rest may have been infected a second time. Recent research is even more compelling, showing that HCV does not return in 99.2 to 100 percent of patients who experience an SVR. French investigators Dr. Sarah Maylin and her colleagues conducted a study of 157 HCV patients who experienced an SVR after treatment, and all of them remained free of the virus four years later. Dr. Maylin and colleagues wrote, "These results strongly suggest that HCV infection is cured in patients who achieve an SVR."[2] In short, once an SVR is reached, HCV is very unlikely to come back.

So, is HCV curable? It absolutely is. In light of that, you might ask, "Why doesn't every HCV patient undergo treatment?" The truth is that there are a few answers to this question, each of which is discussed in this chapter.

> *"We are encouraged . . . because it is rare in the treatment of life-threatening viral diseases that we can tell patients they may be cured."*
>
> —*Mitchell Shiffman, MD, Professor, Virginia Commonwealth University (VCU), Chief of Hepatology and Medical Director of VCU's Liver Transplant Program.*[3]

## WHY SHOULD YOU UNDERGO TREATMENT?

HCV-related cirrhosis is on the rise and expected to peak at 1 million cases by 2020. The rate of HCV-related liver cancer is also increasing, with a projected 14,000 cases annually by 2019. In my opinion, the best way to avoid being one of these devastating statistics is to undergo treatment. HCV medication may permanently eradicate the virus, which means you will live free of the disease. For this reason alone, treatment is worth a try.

Although HCV therapy doesn't guarantee a cure, there are still a number of convincing arguments for its use. HCV patients who respond to treatment report an improved quality of life, even if the response isn't permanent. They feel better, are less fatigued, and have fewer body aches and other HCV-related symptoms. HCV sufferers who receive treatment display improved liver tissue, delayed onset of liver damage, and a reduced chance of cirrhosis, liver cancer, and liver transplantation.

Additionally, HCV therapy can benefit not only your physical well-being but also your mental, social, and spiritual health. In particular, it can help you break free of the stigmas associated with HCV. Patients must often bear the difficult embarrassment of being "infectious," as HCV is a communicable disease. The fear that others have towards you, as well as your fear of infecting others, can be just as difficult to handle as the physical symptoms of HCV. In addition, most HCV sufferers who acquire the virus through drug use are met with an unsympathetic eye from society. This reaction can create guilt and shame, which do nothing but further damage the patient. Each of these stigmas is unnecessarily cruel and difficult to change. Treatment seems to be the best shot at being free of judgment.

Perhaps the greatest benefit that HCV treatment can offer is a sense of personal strength. Since HCV is a chronic disease with an uncertain prognosis, you never know when your condition may change for the worse. It can make you feel helpless. When I went through treatment, I felt like I'd taken back control of my life. I hadn't chosen to get HCV, but I could choose to do something about it. I was about to enter menopause and knew that my chance of beating the virus would drop if I waited any longer. I also knew that I'd regret putting off treatment if things ended up taking a turn for the worse later on. Waiting around for new and better medications seemed like gambling with my life, and I did not want to live with the burden of regret.

# WHAT CAN YOU EXPECT FROM TREATMENT?

Once you understand what to expect from treatment, your decision should become a little easier to make. Knowing which drugs are typically prescribed, how long treatment usually lasts, and what side effects may occur as a result of treatment will surely help sway your internal debate one way or the other so that you can move forward, whatever your choice may be.

*As I've said, the majority of HCV patients will die with and not from this virus. Although this is reassuring, it is not a reason to avoid HCV treatment. The number of people with HCV-related cirrhosis is growing. It's impossible to accurately predict whether or not HCV will progress. Is that a chance you are willing to take with your life?*

## Which Medications Will You Take?

To treat HCV, your medical provider will prescribe medication based on the genotype of your infection. If you have genotype 1, you will likely take a triple therapy combination of peginterferon, ribavirin, and a direct-acting antiviral agent (DAA) such as telaprevir or boceprevir. (See the inset on page 27.) If you have genotype 2 or 3, your provider may recommend using just peginterferon and ribavirin without a third drug. Peginterferon is given by self-injection, usually once a week. The shots don't generally hurt, as they are tiny and go into the fat just below the skin rather than into muscle.

Although it is normal to feel queasy about giving yourself an injection, keep in mind that diabetic children do it several times a day. Even patients who are anxious about it soon master the technique, often reporting that they needn't have worried. Ribavirin is a pill taken orally, usually twice a day. Telaprevir and boceprevir are also taken orally, every eight hours.

# A Few Words About DAAs

Direct-acting antiviral agents (DAAs) offer new hope to HCV sufferers, while potentially adding a new problem to the treatment: drug resistance. A good way to think of DAAs is to compare them to antibiotics. When antibiotics are prescribed, they need to be taken in a designated amount and for a set duration. If the dose or duration is reduced, there's a risk that the bacteria being attacked will not be completely wiped out. Instead, they could adjust to the reduced dose of antibiotic and grow stronger, eventually becoming immune to it. This circumstance would necessitate the use of more powerful medicines, which could create even stronger bacteria. It's a vicious circle that could theoretically happen with HCV DAAs, so always take the medication exactly as prescribed.

Although HCV medications are very expensive, they are covered by most insurance plans. The common forms of peginterferon, Pegasys and PegIntron Redipen, need to be refrigerated, which is also recommended for Victrelis, a brand of boceprevir. I actually know a patient who went on a three-month motorcycle trip through Europe and kept his peginterferon in an insulated cooler. He is now free of HCV and has wonderful travel memories as well.

## How Long Will Treatment Last?

Length of treatment is based on your genotype and initial response to medication. Patients with genotype 2 or 3 can expect twenty-four weeks of treatment, although recent clinical trials have been known to shorten this duration to twelve to sixteen weeks. Treatment length for genotype-1 patients is twenty-four to forty-eight weeks, depending on initial response, with some experts recommending seventy-two weeks for a small subset of genotype-1 patients who do not respond quickly.

## What Are the Side Effects of Treatment?

Although the potential side effects of HCV medication can make you think twice before agreeing to treatment, the range of experiences varies from barely noticeable to intermittently intense. I know patients who climbed 14,000-foot peaks and ran triathlons during treatment, while others could barely drag themselves through a day of work. My experience was fairly typical. I worked a demanding job, traveled extensively, and walked nearly every day. Was it hard? The honest answer is "Yes." Was it the hardest thing I've ever done? Not by a long shot.

When it comes to HCV therapy, it is natural to fear the unknown. But in reality, there is nothing mysterious about interferon, the main drug used against HCV, because it naturally exists in our bodies. It is a protein produced by the immune system, and if you have ever had a cold or flu virus, then you have experienced the typical side effects of interferon. When a virus enters your body, your immune system activates interferon to fight the invader, creating reactions such as fever, chills, muscle and joint aches, fatigue, and malaise, to name the most common. Peginterferon is simply a synthetic version of this naturally occurring protein, so its side effects are similar.

The complete list of HCV therapy's potential side effects is long and includes:

- Abdominal pain
- Anemia
- Anxiety
- Breathing difficulties
- Chills
- Cough
- Decreased appetite
- Depression
- Diarrhea
- Dizziness
- Dry skin
- Fatigue
- Fever
- Hair loss
- Headache
- Insomnia
- Irritability
- Itchiness
- Joint pain
- Low white blood cell count
- Muscle aches
- Nausea
- Rash
- Taste alteration
- Vomiting
- Weight loss

It is important to know, however, that some reactions are much more common than others. For example, you have approximately a 60-percent chance of experiencing fatigue, but your risk of anxiety is only about 10 percent. And while treatment causes most HCV patients to experience the undesirable flu-like symptoms described earlier, these side effects generally occur only after the first few injections, easing up shortly thereafter. (Although, it must be said that a small percentage of HCV patients have flu-like symptoms after the majority of injections.)

The fact is that most HCV patients do not encounter the side effects of treatment all the time. I have never met anyone who suffered with them constantly. Although I have read reports of such accounts online, they seem as rare as the people who don't experience any side effects at all, of whom I've met only two. And for those who meet with reactions on a regular basis, thankfully, there are ways to manage these problems. For instance, if patients have nausea or insomnia, they are given other medications or non-pharmaceutical means to alleviate these issues.

*Whether or not they had an SVR, most people had improved liver biopsy results after HCV treatment.*

Ultimately, research shows that most people endure at least one side effect during HCV therapy. In large clinical trials of current HCV drugs that took place before these treatments reached the market, the dropout rate due to adverse events was 10 to 14 percent. Of all the patients I've worked with, only one has ceased treatment because of intolerable side effects. Although my numbers are merely anecdotal, they are even lower than the clinical trial average, and make me wonder if they are a result of the early intervention, support, and good information that these patients receive.

My personal and professional experiences with HCV treatment have shown me that anxiety about its side effects is usually worse than the actual adverse reactions. For the most part, side effects occur slowly and are intermittent, remaining manageable throughout treatment. If they were all that bad, could more than half a million Americans, not to mention the millions of other HCV sufferers in the world, have successfully completed therapy?

## WHAT ARE THE ODDS THAT TREATMENT WILL WORK?

Understandably, HCV patients want to know what the chances are that treatment will work. The bottom line is that there is every reason to be encouraged by the data on current drug therapies. Statistics, however, are most helpful when they are regarded as trends instead of absolute certainties. For instance, if you ask me how many people have HCV worldwide, I can look at three reputable sources and get three different answers, none of which is technically wrong. The same is true of HCV treatment data. Mark Twain said it best when he stated, "Facts are stubborn, but statistics are more pliable." So, while this section quotes a few numbers, remember to stay focused on the big picture and avoid getting bogged down in details, even if doing so may be difficult at times.

A new triple-drug regimen that uses telaprevir (Incivek), peginterferon alfa-2a (Pegasys), and ribavirin (Copegus) has shown a permanent elimination of HCV at a rate of 79 percent,[4] with that number climbing as high as 95 percent in certain cases. In addition, patients with the genotype 2 or 3 strain of HCV have experienced response rates of 82 percent when treated with only peginterferon and ribavirin in combination.[5]

In fact, your chance of being cured of the virus can depend on a number of factors specific to your case of HCV, the most common of which are:

- **Age.** Patients who are forty years old or younger have higher SVR rates than those who are older than forty.

- **Coinfection or Comorbidity.** The presence of other infections or diseases can negatively influence SVR.

- **Gender.** Females have a slightly better chance of successful treatment than males.

- **IL-28B Gene Variation.** Patients with the CC form of the IL-28B gene experience higher rates of SVR than those with the CT or TT form of this gene.

- **Presence of Cirrhosis.** Patients with bridging fibrosis or cirrhosis experience fewer SVRs than those without these conditions.

- **Race.** African Americans and Latinos display fewer SVRs than Caucasians, while patients of Asian descent show a higher number of SVRs than Caucasians.

- **Viral Load.** Patients with viral loads of 800,000 IU/mL (international units per milliliter) or lower are more likely to respond to therapy than those with viral loads higher than 800,000 IU/mL.

- **Weight.** Patients who weigh 187 pounds or less display better SVR rates than those who weight more than 187 pounds.

Perhaps the best indicators of your likelihood of being cured are response rates—specifically, the extended Rapid Virologic Response (eRVR), which I will simply call "rapid response," and the Early Virologic Response (EVR), which I will simply call "early response." Patients who display no traces of the virus within four weeks of therapy are deemed rapid responders. Rapid response is highly predictive of sustained response. If you experience rapid response, factors such as your genotype, age, and viral load become less relevant, as rapid response is the best possible predictor of a compete elimination of the disease.

An early response means that there is no detectable HCV after the first twelve weeks of treatment. Responding early does not predict an SVR (28 to 35 percent of patients who have an early response will not experience a permanent elimination of the virus), but the absence of an early response is a strong indication that an SVR will not occur. For this reason, early response is known as a "negative predictor of response." Of those who do not achieve an early response, 97 to 100 percent will fail to have an SVR. [6, 7]

A recent trend in medicine known as *response-guided therapy* (RGT) has doctors making recommendations based on a patient's specific reactions to treatment. A hearty, rapid response may result in a shorter treatment than usual. A weak, delayed response may mean a longer treatment, change in drug regimen, or discontinuation of medication until better options become available. As always, talk to your medical provider about the best course of action for you. Thanks to individualized medicine, recent HCV drugs, and new ways of working with older drugs, experts are confident that a cure for HCV is within reach for the majority of those affected.

> *When discussing your response to treatment with your doctor, you may hear the term "log drop." For instance, your provider may want you to have a two-log drop in your viral load in the first 12 weeks of treatment. The simplest way to determine a log drop is to take your viral load and lop off the last digit. In the case of two-log drop, you would lop off the last two numbers, and so on. For example, if your viral load is 1,800,000 IU/mL, then a two-log drop would result in a viral load of 18,000 IU/mL.*

## COMMON REASONS FOR DELAYING TREATMENT

As far as HCV treatment goes, you can try it, refuse it, or wait to see what new drugs will offer. The choice is yours, and because I struggled with the decision, I understand why others do so. Indecision, however, adds an unnecessary layer of discomfort to the whole experience, sometimes to the point of agony. Winston Churchill stated it well when he said, "I never worry about action, but only inaction." While fear is most often responsible for the indecision associated with HCV treatment, there may be a few other factors at work.

### Lack of Consequences

It is wonderful when the decision comes easily, but frequently it doesn't. It didn't for me. I sat on the fence for quite some time. I felt fine, didn't have cirrhosis, had stopped drinking, and was taking decent care of myself. I knew that, statistically speaking, I was more likely to die of a cause other than HCV. In short, I had no compelling reason to try therapy. This same situation confronts a great number of HCV patients. It is hard to make a decision when the consequences of *not* making one aren't pressing down on you, causing you to feel sick. If I had thought that cirrhosis was inevitable, the choice would have been easier to make. Had liver cancer seemed more of a possibility, I would not have thought twice before going ahead with treatment. But I urge you not to let complacency stand in the way of a potential cure for your HCV.

## Distrust of Traditional Medication

A patient used to call me periodically, looking for a holistic cure for HCV. When it came to treatment, she wanted to stick with "natural medicine." As for traditional HCV therapy, she "was not going to put those toxic poisons" into her body. I always listened to her patiently. One day, I told her that I saw HCV drugs as potent, sacred, and healing—no different from the herbs used by shamans to cure illness. A month later, she started HCV treatment. A year later she was free of the virus and became an ardent supporter of traditional therapy. After her recovery, I heard her speak at support group meetings, confessing that her preconceptions of HCV medication had gotten the best of her.

If HCV drugs still concern you, consider the fact that you can usually stop treatment if the side effects prove intolerable. Keep in mind, though, that this strategy may not apply to new drug treatments, such as the DAAs that are starting to be prescribed along with traditional medications peginterferon and ribavirin. DAAs, which specifically target HCV, may cause viral mutations, so once you start them, it is generally best to stay the course, if you can.

## Inconvenience

It is understandable to worry about the impact that HCV therapy might have on both your work life and your personal life. Unfortunately, such worries usually make it seem as though no time is a good time to start treatment. Yes, it may interfere with your work life and your personal life. But the majority of patients I've known were able to maintain a fairly normal work schedule throughout therapy, some at very demanding jobs. In most instances, all it takes is a few minor modifications to your routine. For example, I often took a nice twenty-minute nap in my car when I needed one. And if you are dealing with personal issues, such as planning a wedding or having problems with a loved one, it's best to get these settled before starting treatment.

If you are a woman over thirty-five years old who still wishes to have children, though, choosing a time to start treatment is a little more complicated. You may decide to undergo therapy right away, before you get pregnant, so as not to pass HCV on to your offspring. Delaying pregnancy, however, may make it more difficult to have a child in the future. Alternatively, you might choose to become pregnant, take the small risk (around 5 percent) of passing HCV on to your baby, and simply live with HCV for a while longer. It's a tough and deeply personal decision.

For everyone else, however, the plain truth is that there may never be a perfect time to undergo HCV therapy. You may just have to aim for a less inconvenient time to start the medication. Otherwise, you'll never do it. But make no mistake, going forward with HCV treatment is not a leap of faith. It is a decision. As R. Buckminster Fuller said, "Our power is in our ability to decide." Claim your power and decide what you want to do about your health and future.

*Don't torture yourself with indecisiveness about treatment. Not making a decision is a decision to not undergo treatment.*

## New Drugs

I have known a few people who didn't think twice before starting therapy, and I was curious to know what led to their rapid decisiveness. Most said that they trusted their medical providers and were simply following medical advice. My absolute favorite response came from an HCV patient who said, "I got HCV from using heroin. I didn't ask my drug dealer about *its* side effects or if I should wait for something better. I figure my doctor is more trustworthy than a drug dealer."

As you read this, you may hear about a new HCV medication being researched. Wanting the best treatment, you may assume that the drugs in the pipeline will be worth the wait, but that belief may not turn out to be true. If you're holding off on therapy for this reason, here are a few facts to consider:

❏ At this juncture, the HCV drugs that are on the market provide excellent results.

❏ If you are hoping to avoid peginterferon, it is unlikely that it will be excluded from treatment for some time.

❏ There are always new medications around the bend, but many will not make it to market.

❏ There is no time like the present. HCV treatment is more effective the younger you are.

Talk to your medical provider about the best time and medication for your condition. If a new treatment will soon be available and seems best for you, your doctor may recommend it. On the other hand, if it looks like the newest medications won't be on the market for quite some time, it may be best to start treatment immediately using current drugs, particularly if your disease is advanced. Furthermore, your insurance provider may not cover new, often very expensive drugs, even if they are available. (One way to solve the problems of cost and availability is to try to join clinical trials of a new drug, which typically supply the new medication for free.)

## WHEN IS TREATMENT NOT RECOMMENDED?

Sometimes, even if you would like to pursue HCV treatment, certain conditions make current drug therapy inadvisable. HCV medication is not recommended for patients who:

- are living with untreated thyroid disease that may be worsened by antiviral therapy.

- are pregnant or breastfeeding, or who may become pregnant and are unwilling or unable to comply with effective contraception. In addition, men with HCV who have partners who are pregnant or breastfeeding, or who may become pregnant should not be treated.

- are taking certain substances that may interact with HCV medications, including alfuzosin hydrochloride, anti-seizure drugs, atorvastatin, cisapride, drosperinone-containing drugs, oral midazolam, ergot-containing medicines, lovastatin, pimozide, rifampin, sildenafil citrate, tadalafil, St. John's wort, and triazolam. (See Chapter 5.)

- are younger than two years of age.

- have a serious concurrent medical issue, such as severe hypertension, heart failure, significant coronary artery disease, poorly controlled diabetes, chronic lung disease, or kidney disease.

- have a significant, untreated ophthalmic disorder, such as cotton wool spots.

- have a bacterial infection or blood disorder, such as sickle-cell anemia or thalassemia major.

- have been diagnosed with autoimmune hepatitis or another autoimmune condition known to be exacerbated by HCV medications.

- have decompensated cirrhosis, unless therapy is done under close supervision at a liver transplant center.

- have experienced hypersensitivity to any HCV medication.

- have received certain organ transplants, such as a kidney, heart, or lung transplant. (This recommendation does not include a liver transplant.)

- Suffer with major uncontrolled depression or psychiatric illness.

Tell your medical provider if you have HIV, colitis, hepatitis B, cancer, or a history of mental illness, substance abuse, or sleep problems. These will need to be addressed prior to taking HCV medications. Treatment is generally not advised if you are an active alcoholic or in early recovery.

*Ribavirin is a category X drug, which means it may cause birth defects or death to a fetus. If you are a woman who may become pregnant or a male partner of a fertile woman, rule out pregnancy before beginning HCV treatment. If pregnancy occurs immediately prior to treatment, during treatment, or six months after treatment has stopped, tell your medical provider immediately. All pregnancies should be reported to the Ribavirin Pregnancy Registry, a confidential and free public health program, by either you or your doctor. (See the Resources on page 148.)*

There are, of course, exceptions to these guidelines. Even if one of these conditions applies to you, your HCV may be so serious that your medical provider advises treatment anyway, under close supervision. For example, patients with an autoimmune condition such as rheumatoid arthritis or advanced liver disease have been safely treated for HCV. Additionally, people who are dependent on drugs or using methadone to help ease withdrawal symptoms of opiate drug addiction have been successfully treated by experienced medical providers. Finally, I have worked with quite a few patients who went through HCV treatment after getting their diabetes, depression, heart disease, or thyroid disease under control.

Ultimately, if your medical provider does not advise treatment, it is your responsibility to ask why. If his reasons are sound and you trust him, then no further action is necessary. If you have any doubt, get a second opinion. Remember, though, that the reverse is also true. If a provider advises treatment and you don't think you are a good candidate, get a second opinion.

##  THE BOTTOM LINE

While I generally favor treatment for HCV sufferers, I understand that it may not be for every patient. The choice to pursue drug therapy is a personal one, and should be thoughtfully considered before deciding one way or the other. Simply remember the following points when making your choice.

❑ According to recent research, 99.2 to 100 percent of the time, HCV does not return once a patient experiences an SVR as a result of treatment.

❑ HCV sufferers show improved liver health after treatment, even if they did not respond to the medication.

❑ HCV treatment typically causes moderate side effects, and no one experiences them all the time.

❑ Most side effects are manageable, particularly with early medical intervention.

❑ HCV treatment is more effective the younger you are. If you can do it now, you maximize your chances of responding to the medication.

❑ Fear is not a good reason to avoid treatment.

❑ Patients with certain medical conditions, pregnant women, and the partners of pregnant women should not be treated with current HCV drugs. If you have a condition that makes HCV treatment inadvisable, talk to your doctor and see if getting it under control will allow you to undergo treatment.

Do not, however, allow your thoughtful consideration to turn into harmful indecision. Try HCV therapy or don't try it, but don't spend too much time sitting on the fence, as that precious time could cost you your health.

# — 3 —

# HOW TO MAXIMIZE YOUR HEALTH WHILE YOU CONSIDER HCV TREATMENT

*No time for your health today will result in
no health for your time tomorrow.* —IRISH PROVERB

CV or no HCV, the best advice I have ever received is this: Make health a priority. Good health habits will serve you well whether or not you have the virus, and whether or not you decide to undergo treatment for it. While keeping a close eye on the health of your liver is important, don't focus solely on HCV-related conditions. I have seen far too many patients who concentrated exclusively on their HCV only to develop an unrelated problem. Of the three deaths in my HCV support group, two were unrelated to HCV-related liver disease. The same was true of the patients I worked with at Stanford. Essentially, by maintaining a healthy body, you will be protecting yourself not only from HCV-related liver disease but also from a host of other illnesses.

Remember, though, maintaining wellness is about more than taking care of your body. It includes keeping your mind healthy, too. In this chapter, you will learn how to improve your overall well-being while you consider treatment options for HCV. As self-improvement often involves making significant changes in your life, always remember to be gentle with yourself. Change is more likely to be useful and long-lasting if it is made in small increments rather than large, sweeping ones. The foundation for effective change includes intention, commitment, support, and a reasonable plan. This chapter details the life adjustments that will bring the most benefits to your health.

## AVOID ALCOHOL, CIGARETTES, AND OTHER TOXIC SUBSTANCES

With over 500 functions, the liver is a hardworking organ that processes everything you take in. Whatever you eat, drink, breathe, or absorb through your skin passes through the liver. Although this organ is resilient and remarkable, there are, nevertheless, limits to what it can do. Perhaps the best way to protect the liver is to avoid or reduce the burden placed on it by toxic substances. Alcohol is one of these toxic substances and a major culprit in liver disease— so much so, that even those without HCV can incur liver damage from drinking too much. According to the Hepatitis C Support Project, alcohol consumption:

- accelerates HCV replication

- boosts fat accumulation in and around the liver

- can damage liver cells

- increases iron storage in the liver

- lowers immune system response

- raises risk of viral mutation

- reduces response to HCV treatment

Most medical providers recommend total abstinence from alcohol for their HCV patients. Since alcohol does nothing to improve liver health, it is best to avoid it. HCV patients who do not want to abstain often wonder how much alcohol they can safely drink. There is no guaranteed safe amount. I struggled with the issue of having an occasional drink before deciding to quit. I abstained for five years, but it crept back in after a doctor told me that an occasional glass of wine probably wouldn't hurt me. The word "probably," however, stuck in my head. Every time I drank, I wondered if I was harming my liver, and the worry outweighed the pleasure of the wine. In the end, it was easier for me to give up alcohol than to live in fear that I might be doing damage.

When it comes to mortality rates, more people die from tobacco and illegal drug use than from HCV. These toxic substances not only tax your liver but are destructive to your whole body, and should be given up. I understand, though, that this may be easier said than done. If you want to quit or reduce your use of chemical substances, it is best to do so with help rather than on your own. Thankfully, there are organizations that can aid you in your effort. (See the Resources on page 148.) Unless your doctor advises immediate HCV treatment, I suggest you kick the habit before beginning therapy rather than during it.

In addition to illegal drugs, prescription and over-the-counter medications may cause liver damage, particularly when used other than prescribed. The risks increase when certain drugs are combined. Here are some guidelines to help minimize the chance of harming your liver:

- Always take medication as directed.

- Before taking herbs or supplements, make sure they are compatible with your medication.

- Do not take someone else's medication.

- Inform your medical providers about everything you take, prescribed or not.

- Never mix medications with alcohol and drugs.

- Store medication properly.

*Words from a wise HCV patient: "I view occasional moderate drinking in much the same way as Russian roulette; it's like putting a gun to my liver, pulling the trigger, and hoping I don't shoot myself."*

You may have heard that acetaminophen (Tylenol) is bad for the liver. Unfortunately, the benefits of this drug have been overshadowed by reports of its hazards. Sometimes even well-intended but misinformed medical providers will discourage HCV patients from taking acetaminophen. The truth is that this product is usually safe if taken as directed. The danger comes from taking too much or consuming it with alcohol. Simply ask your physician what the appropriate dosage is for you. Of course, patients with advanced liver disease—particularly those with decompensated cirrhosis—need to be especially careful to follow medical advice before using acetaminophen or other medications.

Chemicals and poisons may also result in liver damage or death. Avoid handling or inhaling potentially noxious substances, such as ammonia, glue, and solvents. When you must use them, learn how to do so safely. Do not breathe in fumes from paints, cleaning products, or other chemicals.

*You are ultimately responsible for your liver. If you are drinking, using drugs, or taking risks with your health by abusing other substances, consider getting some help from a recovery organization or professional. To learn more about these groups and individuals, see the Resources on page 148.*

## USE HERBS, VITAMINS, AND OTHER DIETARY SUPPLEMENTS WISELY

The only proven way to eliminate chronic HCV infection is with medication. Dietary supplements, including herbs, amino acids, vitamins, minerals, and other substances, may help with symptoms but are not effective treatments for complete elimination of the illness. More importantly, it is crucial that you use such products wisely and understand that they can do harm as well as good, especially if you have been diagnosed with HCV.

I have great respect for the value of supplements, but I also have concerns. People sometimes use them because they are "natural," but natural does not mean safe. Since everything passes through the liver, you must be absolutely sure that what you are taking is safe for this organ. Ideally, you should be sure it is safe for your entire body. Herbs are not strictly regulated by the FDA, so it is hard to know what is safe and effective. Truth be told, some people take certain supplements as a result of positive word-of-mouth or because a sales clerk recommended them for liver health. Few actually investigate the safety and effectiveness of herbs any more deeply than that.

If you take supplements, tell your medical provider. Supplements can interact with other medications, have side effects, and may be harmful to your liver or other organs. Apply the same common-sense investigation to dietary supplements as you would to any medicine. For instance, in the same way that you would normally check to see if a new medication might interact with other drugs you are taking, you should also check to see if your new supplements might interact with any drugs or other supplements in your daily routine.

Some supplements are potentially toxic to the liver. Two to watch out for are excess vitamin A and iron. If you take a multivitamin, talk to your medical provider. She may advise you to take a low-iron or no-iron version. If you take vitamin C, use caution, as vitamin C may increase the liver's absorption of iron. When it comes to vitamin A, the beta carotene form of the nutrient is safer than its retinol form, and getting either form through food sources is safer than getting the vitamin through supplements.

Resist all temptation to take large doses of vitamins or other supplements. The body is built to use only what it needs. At best, large doses are eliminated by the body, hurting only your bank account. At worst, high doses may be deadly. While the number of products that may harm the liver is too large to list each one here, the following examples are the most common and potentially toxic supplements.

❑ Any herb containing naturally occurring insecticides called *pyrrolizidine alkaloids*, including borage leaf, coltsfoot, comfrey, and some Chinese medicinal herbs.

❑ Black Cohosh *(Cimicifuga racemosa)*

❑ Chaparral *(Larrea tridentata)*

❑ Germander *(Teucrium chamaedrys)*

❑ Iron

❑ Jin Bu Huan *(Lycopodium serratum)*

❑ Kava *(Piper methysticum)*, also known as kava kava

❑ Niacin, also known as vitamin B$_3$, niacinamide, and nicotinic acid. There have been multiple reports of hepatoxicity when niacin was used in large doses or moderate doses in sustained-release form. But remember, niacin is a necessary nutrient and the Recommended Daily Allowance (RDA) is safe to take.

❑ Pennyroyal *(Hedeoma pulegiodes, Mentha pulegium)*

❑ Skullcap *(Scutellaria lateriflora, S. baicalensis)*

❑ Valerian *(Valeriana officinalis)*

❑ Vitamin A

❑ Yohimbe *(Pausinystalia yohimbe)*

There are plenty of herbs and other supplements that are not specifically toxic to the liver but are nonetheless potentially dangerous to other organs. Some Chinese herbs have been found to contain contaminants such as arsenic, cadmium, lead, mercury (sometimes in the form of calomel or cinnabar), and thallium. Always investigate a supplement carefully before you ingest it, discuss the matter with your physician or pharmacist, and purchase herbs only through reputable sources.

One herb that is particularly popular among HCV patients is milk thistle *(Silybum marianum)*. This flowering plant is native to the Mediterranean but grows all over the world. Milk thistle is believed to protect the liver, and has been used in folk medicine for thousands of years. It has even caught the attention of mainstream research. While the data are inconclusive, milk thistle is generally safe for most people when taken in moderate amounts. (Always be sure, however, to avoid milk thistle products that contain alcohol extracts.) The only real problem with milk thistle is that the version you buy in stores may not be as effective as pharmaceutical grade products. Since the quality of this supplement varies between manufacturers, always purchase a brand from a reputable manufacturer. To fully investigate a product, however, you must learn what to look for in a supplement.

## How to Buy Dietary Supplements

The quality of the vitamins, minerals, and other supplements you buy will have a direct effect on your health. To begin, it's important to know that there are four grades of supplements. From highest-quality to lowest, they are as follows:

❏ **Pharmaceutical grade.** This grade meets the highest regulatory requirements for purity, dissolution (ability to dissolve), and absorption. Pharmaceutical grade supplements are 99-percent pure, with no binders, fillers, dyes, or other unknown substances. Quality is assured by an outside party—the United States Pharmacopeia (USP). This high quality, however, does not come cheap. Pharmaceutical grade supplements can be much more expensive than supermarket supplements and are available only from compounding pharmacies, some health food stores, and doctors' offices. In certain states, a prescription is required to obtain supplements of this quality.

❏ **Medical grade.** These supplements are also high in quality, but may not meet all the standards for purity set by the USP.

❏ **Cosmetic or nutritional grade.** Supplements of this grade are often not tested for purity, dissolution, or absorption, and may not contain the amount of active ingredients listed on the label.

❏ **Feed or agricultural grade.** Supplements of this grade are produced for veterinary purposes and should not be used by humans.

To receive the full benefits of your nutritional supplements, choose pharmaceutical grade products when available. A good health food store usually stocks supplements of several different grades. Simply ask which ones are of pharmaceutical quality. Generally, medical trials are performed using pharmaceutical grade supplements, and dosage recommendations are based on these high-quality products. If you use a product of a lower grade, you may be getting far less of the active ingredient than you need for optimal results. For instance, a pharmaceutical grade omega-3 supplement marked "1,000 mg" actually contains a full 1,000 mg of these fatty acids. If you buy a lower-quality product, however, a capsule marked "1,000 mg" may contain only 600 mg of omega-3s, so you would have to take four times as much to receive the same benefits.

When buying supplements that are not of pharmaceutical grade, you still should look for the highest quality possible. The following guidelines should help you identify the purest and most effective products available:

❏ Look for supplements that contain no preservatives or artificial coloring—nothing but the nutrient itself. Be especially careful to avoid ingredients and fillers to which you have a sensitivity or allergy. Usually, the supplement label of a product will tell you if it contains soybeans, dairy, gluten, or other ingredients that may be problematic.

❏ For greatest effectiveness, choose a formulation and dose that is *bioavailable*, which simply means that more of the supplement is absorbed by your system. Typically, natural forms of nutrients are better absorbed than synthetic forms.

❏ As previously mentioned, some herbal supplements have been found to contain contaminants such as arsenic, lead, mercury, cadmium, and pesticides. To avoid these toxins, look for herbs that have a seal of approval from the United States Pharmacopeia (USP), NSF International, or ConsumerLab.com. These groups test products for label accuracy, lack of contamination, and the ability to dissolve and be absorbed by the body.

❏ Make sure that the supplement is packaged in a container that protects it from the light. Amber-colored glass is the best choice. When you purchase the nutrient, ask if it requires refrigeration.

❏ Choose products that have been vacuum-sealed to preserve freshness. When you puncture the paper seal over the container, you should hear a mild popping sound, indicating that the vacuum has been broken. Always be sure that the product's container has a tamper-proof seal.

> *Herbs and other dietary supplements have the potential to help or harm. Before you take these substances, evaluate them. A link to a drug and supplement interactions checker is provided in the Complementary and Alternative Medicine section in the Resources on page 148.*

## WATCH WHAT YOU EAT

Eating a healthful diet and maintaining an appropriate weight for your height are key elements of staying well. Those who are overweight are less likely to respond to HCV treatment. They are also at risk for non-viral hepatitis caused by fat accumulation in and around the liver. Combine this danger with HCV, and you increase your likelihood of progressing to cirrhosis. Of course, there are many opinions about what constitutes a healthful diet. Some people subscribe to the belief that there are specific HCV diets, but I am not one of them. I think it best to look at heart-healthy nutrition guidelines. Stay abreast of the research and follow current mainstream advice; avoid radical diet advice.

The Mediterranean diet is an example of a sensible way to eat. It is not just a diet; it is a lifestyle. With generous amounts of fresh vegetables and fruit, food is flavored with herbs and spices rather than salt. Fish is consumed at least twice a week, with red meat kept to a minimum. Nuts are eaten regularly in small portions. Olive oil and other healthy fats are used. Meals are eaten slowly, enjoyed with family and friends. Although red wine is typically part of the Mediterranean meal, mineral water with a wedge of lime can be a refreshing substitute. (For more information, see the Resources on page 148.)

I like the suggestions made by Michael Pollan in his book *Food Rules: An Eater's Manual*, in which he states, "Eat Food. Not too much. Mostly plants." If you are wondering what Pollan means by "eat food," this is simply his way of urging you to eat *real* food, such as fresh fruit and vegetables, rather than food that has been processed and packaged with ingredients that cannot be identified in nature. In addition to these guidelines, I have a few more suggestions, including:

- Avoid excess sugar, sodium, saturated fat, and trans fatty acids.

- Beware of products that make wild claims, such as herbs and supplements that promise weight loss without diet or exercise.

- Choose low-fat or vegetable-based proteins.

- Do not eat more calories than you use unless you need to gain weight.

- Drink an adequate amount of water. (See page 101.)

- Eat lots of fruit, vegetables, and fiber.

- Follow a healthful food plan that you can live with and maintain.

- Read food labels and check ingredient lists.

- Skip deprivation. Deprivation may be endured for short periods, but it usually results in unhealthful food binges.

- Thoroughly wash produce before eating. (If you can afford it, eat organically grown foods that have not been sprayed with pesticides.)

- Whenever possible, opt for whole, or unrefined, foods, such as brown rice, whole wheat bread, and chickpeas.

As for liver-specific food recommendations, avoid wild, foraged mushrooms (not the kinds served in restaurants or sold in stores). These mushrooms may be poisonous and can injure the liver, leading to liver transplantation or even death. Tragedy has struck more than one family as a result of accidental ingestion of toxic mushrooms. In addition, do not eat raw or undercooked shellfish, though it is fine to eat cooked crab, cooked clams, and other cooked shellfish. The reason to avoid raw shellfish is because of a bacterium called *Vibrio vulnificus*, which is a microorganism that can cause severe liver damage and death. If you must handle raw shellfish, always be cautious. Wear gloves, wash your hands, and be sure to clean everything that comes in contact with shellfish thoroughly, including utensils and surface areas. Do not swim or wade into warm salt water, where Vibrio vulnificus is often found, as it can enter the body through swallowed water or open wounds.

## EXERCISE REGULARLY

Regular exercise is an essential part of keeping fit. It lessens the effects and discomfort of arthritis, osteoporosis (bone loss), back pain, diabetes, depression, and cardiovascular disease. It improves sleep, reduces stress, and enhances your immune system. In addition to burning calories, exercise can improve your energy level, flexibility, balance, muscle tone, strength, and stamina. Simply put, exercise is good for you. That being said, it is not useful to tell someone who is tired and doesn't like to exercise that she needs to exercise. You might as well tell her to climb Mount Everest. I was extremely fatigued for many years, so I avoided physical activity. Eventually I realized that I was tired because I didn't exercise or eat well. But I also learned that making a radical change wasn't effective for me. Instead, I made small changes, and eventually, exercise became part of my daily routine.

Walking is great exercise because it doesn't require anything more than a good pair of shoes, sunscreen, and a safe place to walk. If inclement weather or extreme temperatures are an issue, malls or large stores can provide a comfortable place to walk. Dancing is also good, because it doesn't feel like exercise. Gardening, bicycling, swimming, yoga, Pilates, and tai chi are other fun ways to stay fit. When done regularly, physical fitness is invigorating. To help you with your choice of exercise, you can find numerous fitness programs on television, at libraries, in video stores, and online. More information about physical fitness can be found in the Resources on page 148.

Always talk to your medical provider before starting a new fitness routine. When you are ready to begin, be sensible. Start gradually, stay well hydrated, don't exercise in extreme heat, and use sunscreen when in direct sunlight. Stop exercising if you are injured, and seek medical advice when appropriate. If it has been a while since you've exercised, sore muscles may occur. Apply hot or cold packs, along with gentle stretching or massage. Do not exercise when ill.

## GET ENOUGH SLEEP

Good sleep is the foundation on which all other healthful habits rest. The National Sleep Foundation recommends seven to nine hours of sleep per night. Based on this recommendation, the average American is sleep-deprived. If I am tired, I don't handle stress as well and tend to reach for high-sugar comfort food. I am tempted to slack off on my exercise, telling myself that I am too tired. Such a lapse in caring for my well-being can create a vicious circle if I don't get a good night's sleep and maintain other health-promoting habits.

Sleep problems may take on a life of their own. If you are currently dealing or have ever dealt with the issue, you know it can make you feel like a zombie. The desire for sleep can become an obsession. If you have problems sleeping, discuss this matter with your medical provider. The sooner you get help for sleep issues, the better. For now, try the following techniques to promote good sleep habits.

❏ Ban the television and computer from the bedroom.

❏ Keep your bedroom slightly cool but comfortable.

❏ Establish a regular bedtime and routine.

❏ Engage in quiet, relaxing activities an hour or two before bedtime.

❏ Listen to relaxation recordings before retiring.

❏ Make your bedroom a worry-free zone. If you feel the need to worry, tell yourself that you will fret only in the daytime. Learn relaxation techniques to reduce stress and anxiety. (See "Reduce Stress" on page 53.)

❏ Sleep in a room that is dark and noise free. If necessary, use eye shades and earplugs to achieve this atmosphere.

❏ Do not lie awake in bed for more than twenty to thirty minutes. Get up and do something boring for a little while and then go back to bed.

❏ Avoid alcohol, tobacco, and caffeine late in the day.

❏ Do not eat a large meal before bedtime or go to bed hungry.

❏ Your bed is for sleep and sex. To perform all other activities, stay out of bed.

> *Sleep apnea and other sleep-related problems can cause some of the same symptoms that HCV does. Before blaming fatigue and other ailments on HCV, rule out other causes, such as sleep disorders. Links to more information about sleep may be found in the Resources section on page 148.*

## GET VACCINATED

Ben Franklin said, "An ounce of prevention is worth a pound of cure." Immunization is an excellent way to prevent serious medical problems. Since HCV affects the liver, it is important to avoid other liver diseases, such as hepatitis A and hepatitis B. Talk to your medical provider about hepatitis A and B immunizations. Thankfully, it is safe to be vaccinated during HCV treatment, so don't worry if you've already begun therapy. While you are at it, make sure you are current on all your immunizations, including a flu shot.

*The best time to get immunized is now.*

## MAINTAIN YOUR BRAIN

Some patients with HCV report mild cognitive impairment. They call it *brain fog*, although this is not a medical term. Brain fog is completely different from the type of dementia known as hepatic encephalopathy, which occurs with advanced liver disease. Brain fog is frustrating but not serious. It basically feels like you're trying to think and move while trapped in a thick cloud. When I experience it, I don't fight it. Short walks, fresh air, extra sleep, and good hydration help.

Studies that look at patients with Alzheimer's or other conditions that affect cognition show that the brain is like a muscle. In other words, use it or lose it. Although no research has focused specifically on the use of brain-fitness tools as a means of improving the cognitive function of HCV patients, some use them nonetheless. Exercising, doing crossword puzzles, playing a musical instrument, or learning a new language are all good ways to sharpen your brain. For more ideas, see the Resources on page 148.

Finally, list everything you have to gain from treatment. Use this list as a reminder during the foggy days. It is important to remember your goal, especially when you cannot see it.

## NURTURE YOUR MIND

Keeping your body in good shape is undoubtedly important, particularly when you have HCV. But even if you stay fit and follow all the recommendations previously listed in this chapter, a troubled mental state can drastically diminish your overall well-being. So don't focus only on the physical part of your health. Your mindset has a lot more to do with wellness than you realize. Joining support groups, learning relaxation techniques, fostering optimism, and embracing your spirituality are all choices that can work wonders for you, helping you remain healthy in a way that physical routines on their own cannot.

## Find Support

One of the first pieces of advice I give to HCV patients is to join an HCV support group. A good support group is a great place to learn how to live well with this virus. Patients who attend groups and have had HCV for a while often know how to manage symptoms. If they have been through HCV treatment, they can share their experience. They will likely know who the best doctors are, who to avoid, and what resources are available in the community. Communing with other HCV sufferers can make you better informed, and improve your mindset and confidence dramatically.

## Reduce Stress

In some cases, people need more than the support provided by groups. If you are feeling the burden of stress, irritability, depression, anger, or insomnia, or are having trouble concentrating, talk to a medical professional. Health conditions such as thyroid or cardiovascular disease may be causing symptoms that feel like stress or anxiety. If you want further support, consult a psychiatrist, psychologist, or other behavioral health specialist. Counseling can provide a shortcut through hard times.

*Regular physical activity is the best way to prevent brain deterioration.*

Assuming there is no medical cause for your stress, learn how to reduce it or manage it. Relaxation and stress management are life skills that will serve your body, mind, and spirit. There are many techniques, including yoga, tai chi, and qigong, so find what works for you. Meditation is an effective relaxation technique for me. At first, I resisted it because I couldn't sit still. It was frustrating to meditate while my brain was chattering away about all sorts of things. I'd get restless and quit, but I stuck with it because I wanted more peace in my life. Eventually, as I grew calmer and my mind became clearer, I could feel it working.

There are many ways to meditate. One simple method is to find a quiet room, free of external distraction, and sit in a comfortable position, resting your hands on your lap. Gently close your eyes. Inhale through your nose and notice the feeling of the air as it passes through your nostrils and into your lungs, and the expanse of your belly. Think, "Breath in, one." Exhale through your mouth, noticing the air as it leaves your lungs and mouth. Think, "Breath out, one." Do this again, this time thinking, "Breath in, two." Exhale and think, "Breath out, two." Continue doing this until you reach the count of ten, all the while noticing your breathing. When you reach ten, begin again.

You can do this type of meditation for as long as you like. I suggest starting with five minutes and building to twenty minutes. If your mind wanders, simply bring it back to the breathing, and count from wherever you left off or begin again at one. It gets easier with practice. Throughout your day, if you notice that you are feeling stressed, take a moment to concentrate on your breathing. It's amazing how much relief a few focused breaths will bring.

Ultimately, it is easier to stay relaxed if you don't overcommit yourself in life. Learn to set limits and say no to requests that you do not want to fulfill. Taking care of yourself means knowing when to rest, when to work, and when to play. "To thine own self be true" is a good motto to put into practice.

## Maintain a Positive Attitude

In addition to learning stress-reduction skills, do your best to maintain a positive attitude. I used to bristle when I heard people tell HCV patients to, "keep a positive attitude; practice gratitude; say affirmations, and so on," as if we could just think our way to health. But the evidence and spirit of others compelled me to keep an open mind. Eventually, I traded in skepticism and misery for a positive attitude. Either way, I still have HCV, but it is easier to live with the disease when I take an optimistic approach to life.

Developing a positive attitude is a lifelong process. Start by considering your thoughts. Don't judge them; just notice them. Perhaps you entertain thoughts such as, "I'll never feel good," "I am exhausted," "I hate feeling this way," "My life is ruined," or "HCV is killing me." After you notice these ideas, experiment with an alternative, more positive perspective. Try, "I am learning how to feel good," "I am getting my energy back," "I am getting stronger," "I am grateful to be alive," or "My liver is amazing." Pretty soon, you won't just be saying these statements, you'll believe them.

If you're having trouble moving your mind in the right direction, find some inspiration. I am inspired by the strength and courage of others, particularly the HCV patients I've worked with. After cancer survivor Lance Armstrong made his comeback in the cycling world, one of my patients told me that she would never complain about having HCV again. Another inspiring star is Zimbabwean singer Prudence Mabhena. Deformed and legless due to a congenital disease, she nevertheless launched an amazing music career. And there is Dan Caro, a drummer, author, and motivational speaker who nearly died after being burned at the age of two. Dan says, "When you change the way you look at things, the things you look at change." There is no shortage of positive people out there. Surround yourself with them and you'll be thinking positively in no time.

*Positive thinking can complement any type of healing art. The way I look at it, living with a positive attitude feels better than living with a negative one.*

## Consider Spirituality

Spirituality and religion are deeply personal matters, and for that reason I will say little about them. Spiritual belief is central to the lives of some, however, and not mentioning this fact in a book about healing is like talking about automobiles without discussing fuel. If you believe in the power of prayer or faith healing, employ these tools as you find useful. Personally, I found it helpful to view the treatment process as healing not just my liver but my whole self, including my spirit.

If you don't feel comfortable with the spiritual side of life, perhaps you might respond to the power of nature. For a few minutes each day, try sitting in a place you consider beautiful. Alternatively, you can simply imagine the place, whether it be on a beach, beside a flowing river, on a mountain top, or in a lush forest. Any method that works for you is worth practicing, whether or not you plan to pursue therapy.

## THE BOTTOM LINE

Medical care is necessary to eliminate HCV; make no mistake about that. This does not mean, however, that every HCV patient opts for treatment. While you consider therapy, the best thing you can do is focus on physical and mental fitness. As you attempt to make a decision, remember the following points.

❏ Health is more than taking care of just the body. Optimal health includes body, mind, and spirit.

❏ A positive attitude and a reduction in stress levels are powerful companions to any physical health regimen.

❏ Support and counseling are valuable tools in the maintenance of your well-being.

❏ Physical activity can alleviate both physical and psychological problems.

❏ Whatever you eat, drink, breathe, or absorb through your skin passes through the liver, including toxins.

❏ Look for evidence that a drug or dietary supplement will work before you use it as treatment.

❏ Some herbs and supplements can cause liver damage, so be careful when considering such products.

❏ Immunization can prevent you from getting certain forms of hepatitis as well as some other diseases.

Ultimately, a healthy body will help stave off not only HCV-related illnesses but also a multitude of other health conditions. A positive and relaxed mental state will provide a solid foundation for you to get through the hard days and various psychological issues that accompany a diagnosis of HCV. Combined with the medical treatment, the techniques outlined in this chapter can offer powerful therapy for the disease.

# —4—

# How to Prepare for and Begin HCV Treatment

*Well begun is half done.* —ARISTOTLE

I f you have decided to go ahead with treatment, you may feel a mixture of relief and anxiety, which is perfectly normal. With the decision out of the way, though, it is time to move forward. Hopefully, you took the advice given in Chapter 3 and have been strengthening your body, mind, and spirit while you were considering HCV therapy. There is now, however, more work to be done. From checking your insurance coverage and becoming familiar with your prescribed drugs to learning how to take your medication and establishing a routine, there are ways to make the process of destroying the HCV virus run smoothly. This chapter outlines where your focus should lie as you prepare for and begin HCV therapy.

## CHECK YOUR COVERAGE

HCV treatment is very expensive. The Fair Pricing Coalition estimates the cost of a twelve-week supply of just the DAA telaprevir (Incivek) to be approximately $49,200. Treatment with the DAA boceprevir (Victrelis), which requires twenty-four weeks worth of medication, amounts to around $22,000, while combination therapy that uses only peginterferon and ribavirin is priced at about $15,000. Factor in the price of medical appointments, lab tests, and drugs to manage side effects and you end up with bills that few can afford without medical insurance. In light of these facts, you should check your insurance coverage before you begin treatment. Do you have prescription coverage? If so, what will your out-of-pocket costs be? How often will you need to see your medical provider and get lab tests done, and what will your co-pays be? Do you have any reason to think that your medical insurance will stop during treatment, such as a potential job layoff? If so, will you be able to afford insurance premium payments? These are all questions that need to be answered.

> *If your HCV drugs are covered, determine your co-pay. It may not be the same as your regular co-pay amount, as some companies cover injectable drugs under a different portion of the policy. Your regular prescription co-pay should apply for oral drugs such as ribavirin, telaprevir, and boceprevir.*

If the required drugs are not covered by your plan, see if you qualify for financial aid. Most drug companies have assistance programs for low-income uninsured and underinsured patients. Contact each drug manufacturer online or by phone before filling your prescriptions, as these programs can offer substantial savings. In addition, choosing the generic form of a drug may also reduce the cost of treatment. For example, the generic version of ribavirin sells for about half of what the brand name costs. Unfortunately, newer medications such as telaprevir and boceprevir may not have generic equivalents for quite some time. Finally, shop around for low prices, which can sometimes be found at well-known Internet-based pharmacies or bulk chains, such as Costco and Sam's Club.

If, despite trying the previous budget-minded measures, price puts HCV treatment out of reach, see if you qualify for a clinical trial. Usually, these are offered at major medical centers, but some smaller medical offices may also be used as test sites. Ask your medical provider about clinical trials in your area.

## TALK TO YOUR MEDICAL PROVIDER ABOUT TREATMENT

Talking to your medical provider is a great way to get information about HCV treatment. A good doctor or nurse should welcome your questions. Nevertheless, even if you see the most receptive physician there is, office visits last only a certain amount of time. You can use your time more effectively if you write down your questions and prioritize them before your appointment. At the beginning of the visit, tell your provider that you have a list of questions that you'd like to ask. Doing so should allow her to manage the time accordingly. If you still have questions by the end of the visit, ask your provider to suggest a way to have them answered outside the office.

Here are some issues you may want to discuss before starting HCV treatment:

- **Antidepressants.** Be sure to tell your provider if you take antidepressants or have a history of depression. As HCV medication can cause depression, some physicians recommend a psychiatric consultation prior to starting treatment. If you are not already taking an antidepressant, one may be prescribed for you. Most antidepressants take two to four weeks to become effective, but some take six to eight weeks. Besides depression, antidepressants may help alleviate treatment-induced side effects such as fatigue, anxiety, insomnia, and pain. They may also, however, produce their own side effects, including decreased libido, or sex drive. There are many antidepressants from which to choose, so discuss them with your medical provider. Finally, never take any over-the-counter dietary supplement for depression without talking to your doctor first. (See "Dietary Supplements" below.)

- **Birth Control.** If there is even a remote possibility of pregnancy, be sure you are protected. This also applies to female partners of men on HCV treatment.

- **Dietary Supplements.** If you presently take any supplements, or wish to take a supplement to alleviate a side effect of treatment, discuss the matter with your doctor, who may prohibit the use of certain substances during HCV therapy. For example, St. John's wort, which some people use as an antidepressant, should never be combined with therapy that includes boceprevir or telaprevir. Some doctors, however, recommend taking iron-free multivitamins, calcium, and vitamin D supplements during treatment.

- **Emergencies.** Find out which reactions your medical provider considers emergencies, and how you might reach her if an emergency arises when the office is closed.

- **Length of Treatment.** As previously mentioned, one of the most exciting developments in HCV treatment is the use of response-guided therapy (RGT), which may shorten the length of your program. (See page 31.) Ask your provider if RGT will be used.

- **Medical Procedures.** If you have an upcoming medical or dental procedure planned, check with your doctor to see if it is advisable to undergo before or during HCV treatment.

- **Medication.** Take note of the names and dosages of your prescribed drugs, the methods of administering them, and the estimated length of treatment. Ask if you will receive prefilled syringes or another type of delivery system, and see if you can get a starter kit at your doctor's office. Otherwise, get one from the pharmaceutical company.

- **Schedules.** Inquire about the schedule of regular medical appointments, lab tests, and pregnancy tests.

- **Side Effect Management.** Ask your physician if it is safe to take over-the-counter drugs such as acetaminophen (Tylenol) for your flu-like side effects. If it is, be sure to learn how often you can take them, as well as their recommended dosages.

- **Support.** If you have non-emergency questions or issues that you would like addressed in between appointments, ask your doctor what the best way to handle them might be. Find out if there are any HCV support groups in your community.

Treatment may feel overwhelming at times, particularly since it is uncharted territory. At first, it will sound as though your health practitioner is speaking a foreign language. If you can, take notes during your office visit and bring along a trusted friend or family member. Studies show that no matter how hard patients try, they don't accurately hear all the information their medical providers give them. An extra set of ears can compensate for this problem. If your doctor allows it, you might even record your appointment.

It is your medical provider's job to keep you safe, but she cannot do her job if you don't talk to her. Always keep in mind that small problems are easier to handle than big problems. Discuss your concerns before they get out of hand.

*Some pharmaceutical companies offer starter kits for their drugs. The starter kit I received had an informative video, cooler, pill organizer, band-aids, a container for used needles, and other helpful items.*

## HAVE A COMPLETE MEDICAL EVALUATION

By the time you are given the green light to begin HCV treatment, any of your other medical issues should already have been addressed. As you read in the previous chapter, conditions such as diabetes, major depression, and thyroid disease must be brought under control before starting therapy. Your medical provider will order tests to determine the status of your health and the best course of action for your situation. The following list details each of these tests.

- **Baseline Lab Tests.** These tests consist of a complete blood count (CBC), blood chemistry (including liver tests), and thyroid test.

- **Baseline Physical Exam.** This exam involves checking your weight and blood pressure, as well as other general assessments. Your weight determines the dosages of your medication.

- **Cardiac Evaluation.** If you are older than fifty or have a history of heart disease, your provider may order this evaluation.

- **Eye Exam.** The eye exam is often overlooked. Although the risk for serious eye problems is low, it is advisable to have a baseline eye exam prior to treatment.

- **Genotype.** This test determines which strain of HCV you have, which determines how long you will require treatment.

- **Immunizations.** Your provider will verify that all your immunizations are current, including those for hepatitis A and B, flu, and tetanus. It is permissible to get these shots during treatment, if necessary.

- **Pregnancy Test.** You should not start treatment if there is any possibility that you are pregnant.

- **Viral Load (HCV RNA).** This test measures the amount of HCV in your blood and may influence the length of treatment, especially when compared with results after you start therapy.

Additionally, you will need to attend medical visits and have lab work done regularly throughout treatment. The schedule varies among providers, but typically patients are seen a week or two after they start therapy, and then every month after that for the first twelve weeks. The intervals between appointments may be longer towards the end of treatment, increasing to between eight and twelve weeks, assuming both the patient and provider are comfortable with this arrangement and have a reliable way to communicate lab results and other concerns. As previously mentioned, some newer treatment regimens include response-guided therapy, in which a patient's viral loads are monitored more frequently and treatment is adjusted according to the results.

## FOLLOW YOUR DRUG PROTOCOL

As you know, HCV treatment consists of either triple-drug therapy or combination therapy, depending on which strain of the virus you have. It involves taking drugs orally and by injection at designated intervals. The sooner you become familiar with HCV medication protocol, the sooner you will rid yourself of any anxiety or confusion over the process.

## Obtaining Your Medication

First, don't expect to get a prescription, walk into your local drugstore, and leave with the medication that day. These drugs are extremely expensive, and most insurance companies require prior approval. Additionally, some pharmacies don't keep these medications on hand and will need to order them. In some cases, your insurance company may require you to use a specialty pharmacy, which will ship the drugs directly to you. If you pick up your medication at your local pharmacy, remember to bring a cooler and ice pack with you to safely transport any drugs that require refrigeration.

*It is important to rule out pregnancy before beginning HCV treatment. Additionally, patients should wait six months from the date of their last pill and shot before attempting to become pregnant. If pregnancy occurs immediately prior to the end of treatment, during treatment, or six months after treatment has stopped, tell your medical provider right away. All pregnancies should be reported to the Ribavirin Pregnancy Registry. (See the Resources on page 148.)*

## Starting Treatment

Plan to begin your therapy with an evening injection, unless your medical provider wants you to do the first injection in the office. If you work a typical work week schedule, Friday evening is a good time to start treatment, as it gives you the weekend to recover from initial side effects. We all have our own priorities, though. One patient I knew preferred to administer his injections on Sunday evenings so that he'd be at his best when the weekend rolled around.

## Injections

Your medical provider will show you how and where (either your stomach or upper leg) to inject your interferon. The injections aren't painful, but you may feel a slight sting or pinch. Good technique will help you eliminate this issue. When administering your shot, remember these points:

❏ Gather your supplies. You will need instructions, alcohol wipes, a sharps container (a canister designed to collect your used syringes and needles), your medication, and needles with syringes.

❏ Wash your hands before taking your medication.

❏ If you are taking the Pegasys or PegIntron Redipen brand of peginterferon, take it out of the refrigerator shortly before your injection so it can come to room temperature.

❏ Prepare your peginterferon in a clean, distraction-free, well-lit place.

❏ After you swab the injection site, let the alcohol evaporate for a few seconds. Doing so reduces the sting of the shot.

❏ Hold the barrel of the syringe like a throwing dart. Take a deep breath, exhale, and aim the needle. Count to three and perform the injection.

❏ After your injection, make sure to activate the needle's safety system. Never reuse a needle or syringe.

❏ Properly dispose of the needle and syringe in your approved sharps container. (These containers can be returned to your pharmacy, medical provider, or community collection service.)

❏ Plan on rotating injection sites to prevent skin damage. Red, blotchy skin at the injection site is common and may last a month or more. If you are a woman and plan on swimming during treatment, you may want to relegate your injections to your stomach and wear a one-piece bathing suit. Men may want to inject into their thighs and wear long swim trunks.

*If you are clean and sober but have a history of intravenous drug use, you may have some apprehension about injecting your HCV medication. Understandably, you may be concerned that the rituals that accompany HCV therapy injections might trigger a relapse. Fortunately, relapse for this reason is uncommon, probably because the injection technique is so different. As previously described, peginterferon is injected into the layer of fat beneath the skin rather than into a vein, and no tourniquet is used. If this method still concerns you, talk to others who have been through treatment. You may hear remarkable insight. As one former drug user with HCV observed, "The needle gave me this disease, and now it will get rid of it."*

Some people find the first injection easier than subsequent ones. Strangely, I hit a wall after the first month, and my hand would stop just before the needle made contact. The shots didn't hurt, and they were easy to give, so I was baffled. I finally realized that I was thinking about it too much. I decided to distract myself by tapping my toes while administering the injection. If I injected in my leg, I'd tap the toes of my opposite foot. This minor distraction helped me until the shots became effortless.

According to the drug's instructions, before administering the shot, it is important to avoid pulling back on the syringe, as doing so may result in injecting the interferon into a vein instead of the fat below the skin. Interferon manufacturers are required by law to give you this warning. Although the information is worthwhile, don't be needlessly afraid of hitting a vein or capillary. It won't hurt you if you do. Moreover, hitting a vein is actually quite difficult to do if you are injecting into your stomach or thighs. Aim for a clear part of your skin where there aren't obvious veins and you should have no problem. In addition, manufacturers warn against having air bubbles in the syringe. Truthfully, though, air bubbles won't hurt you either. They may simply cause a reduced amount of interferon in the syringe. So don't worry if you can't get rid of a tiny bubble. In all the years I have been working with HCV patients, I have never heard of anyone being harmed by an air bubble.

You must refrigerate both the Pegasys and PegIntron brand of peginterferon that comes premixed in the Redipen delivery system. Neither should not be stored in the freezer or left out of the refrigerator for more than twenty-four hours. Unmixed PegIntron that comes in a vial, however, does not need refrigeration.

## Oral Drugs

Unless otherwise directed, you should take ribavirin twice daily with food. Try to take ribavirin with food that has some fat in it, as fat seems to increase absorption of the drug. While you will not harm yourself by taking the medication without food, patients often state that combining it with a meal helps reduce the chance of nausea. If you aren't hungry, try to eat something small, such as yogurt or a piece of cheese.

If you are prescribed a direct-acting antiviral agent (DAA) such as telaprevir or boceprevir, you will take two or four pills, three times a day, seven to nine hours apart. Telaprevir needs to be taken within thirty minutes of eating food that contains at least twenty grams of fat. Boceprevir should be taken with a general meal or light snack. Boceprevir must be refrigerated, but may be stored at room temperature (of no more than 77°F) for up to three months.

## Drug Interactions

As an HCV patient, it is crucial to become familiar with the list of medications that interact poorly with HCV drugs. If you are taking peginterferon and ribavirin without a DAA, this list is relatively short and includes:

- azathioprine *(Azasan, Imuran)*

- methadone *(Dolophine, Methadose)*

- nucleoside reverse transcriptase inhibitors *(NRTI)*, including didanosine *(Videx)* and zidovudine *(Retrovir)*

- telbivudine *(Tyzeka)*

- theophylline *(Aerolate III)*

*As new HCV treatments appear, more medications may be added to the list of drug interactions. Always check with your medical provider or pharmacist prior to taking any drug or supplement.*

The list of drug interactions grows considerably when HCV therapy includes the DAAs boceprevir or telaprevir. You should not take boceprevir or telaprevir with any of these substances:

- alfuzosin hydrochloride *(Uroxatral)*

- anti-seizure medicine such as carbamazepine *(Carbatrol,Tegretol)*, phenobarbital *(Luminal)*, and phenytoin *(Dilantin)*

- atorvastatin *(Lipitor, Caduet)*

- cisapride *(Propulsid)*

- drospirenone-containing medicine *(Yaz, Zarah, Safyral)*

- ergot-containing medicine *(Migranal, Ergotrate, Cafergot, Methergine)*

- lovastatin *(Advicor, Altoprev, Mevacor)*

- midazolam *(Versed)*, when taken orally

- pimozide *(Orap)*

- rifampin *(Rifadin, Rifamate, Rifater)*

- sildenafil citrate *(Revatio)* or tadalafil *(Adcirca)*

- simvastatin *(Zocor, Vytorin, Simcor)*

- triazolam *(Halcion)*

While drospirenone and anti-seizure drugs are contraindicated solely for boceprevir, and atorvastatin is contraindicated only for telaprevir, the rest of the previously mentioned restricted drugs apply to both DAAs. In addition, certain dietary supplements, including St. John's wort and bupleurum, should not be combined with HCV treatment. The majority of dietary supplements, in fact, has not been well tested in connection with HCV therapy and should be approached with caution. If you are taking any substance at all, talk to your doctor before beginning treatment. Personally, I did not want to take any chances while being treated, so the only herbal supplements I used were ginger to help with nausea and various teas to help with other mild symptoms.

## Missing a Dose

Never beat yourself up for missing a dose. If you forget to take your DAA, simply do so when you remember, provided you have more than two hours before your next dose. If you have less than two hours before your next dose, skip the missed dose. Never double up on your DAA. If you neglect to take your ribavirin and there are more than six hours before your next dose, it is usually safe to go ahead and take your pills. If there are less than six hours, simply wait for your next dose to get back on schedule. Never double up on ribavirin, as doing so increases the risk of nausea and vomiting. It's all right to miss a few doses over the long haul, but the fewer you miss, the better.

> *Always read the patient information*
> *included with your medication.*

If you miss your peginterferon injection but less than two days have passed since you were supposed to take it, administer it right away and maintain your regular schedule for shots. If it has been more than two days, you may need to create a new schedule. Speak to your doctor should this occur. In regard to any HCV drug, do not stop taking your medication, switch brands, reduce your dosage, or deliberately skip a dose unless advised to do so by your medical provider.

*Your local pharmacy is another source of support. Pharmacists can answer questions related to your medication.*

## Getting Support from Drug Companies

Your medical provider is the expert you pay to take care of you. You may be afraid, however, of asking her too many questions and seeming like a "pain in the neck." I urge you to let go of this fear. This is your health, not a popularity contest. Of course, even if you are very comfortable with your physician, questions can still pile up in your mind. It's often difficult to gauge the seriousness of certain issues. Should you wait until your next appointment for answers, or should you call immediately? You may wish you had a direct hotline to your provider. Fortunately, there are other sources that offer support.

Drug companies that sell HCV pharmaceuticals often provide free programs to help you get your questions answered. These toll-free telephone service lines are offered around the clock, seven days a week, and feature nurses who address your queries. Depending on the company, you may talk to a live person, or you may leave a detailed message, to which a nurse will respond within thirty minutes to a couple of hours.

In addition to phone support, these programs can remind you to take your medication via email, provide excellent web-based resources, and send you a starter kit. For those without Internet access, information can be mailed to your home. Some companies even offer classes to show you how to administer the medication. In rural areas, they will conduct these classes in your home or provider's office. All of these services are confidential.

*Make a habit of storing your keys, wallet, purse, checkbook, mobile phone, and other such items in the same place each day. It's easy enough to lose track of their location on a good day, let alone when you're dealing with HCV treatment.*

## CREATE A ROUTINE

HCV drugs must be taken in certain doses and at certain times—a fact that makes organization critical to success. This is particularly true of DAAs, which, as you know, carry the risk of creating drug-resistant HCV variants when not taken as directed. Treatment consists of injecting peginterferon once a week, swallowing ribavirin pills twice a day, and, if triple-drug therapy is prescribed, taking two or four DAA pills every seven to nine hours. Advising you to follow your prescriptions may seem obvious and unnecessary, but side effects such as fatigue and insomnia can lead to forgetfulness, which sets the stage for a missed dose or two. As a nurse, I was able to keep track of complicated drug regimens for my patients, but would occasionally neglect my own. I knew that my chance of beating HCV depended on my dedication to therapy, so I discovered ways to keep myself on track.

While undergoing treatment, it is best to maintain a routine in connection with your medication. For example, I took my pills with breakfast and dinner. Thankfully, there are a number of helpful tools that can keep you on a schedule. Do yourself a favor and use a:

❏ calendar to keep track of your injections, appointments, and side effects.

❏ free online service to send yourself email medical reminders or notes of encouragement. (See the Resources on page 148.)

❏ small notepad to jot down thoughts you'd like to discuss with your medical provider.

❏ weekly pill organizer. One may come with your starter kit. The best organizers have two compartments per day, for morning and evening doses.

## PREPARE FOR YOUR MEDICAL APPOINTMENTS

You will receive the full benefit of your medical appointments if you have all your relevant information on hand. To avoid time-wasting searches, keep and update a document with the information listed below and bring it to each office visit.

❏ All recent lab results that screen for other diseases or conditions

❏ Allergies

❏ Current concerns

❏ Family medical history

❏ Immunization records

❏ Information about your HCV, including your genotype, viral load, dates and results of liver biopsies, and dates of past treatment

❏ Medications, including supplements and over-the-counter drugs

❏ Ongoing medical problems

❏ Prescription refills to request from your medical provider

❏ Surgeries

> *You can't control your HCV genotype, viral load, age, or any other factor that affects your chance of permanently eliminating the virus, but you can control the diligence with which you approach therapy.*

## KEEP RECORDS

Always ask for copies of your lab results and other diagnostic tests, which you can use to chart your progress. (See the inset on page 74.)

# Interpreting Lab Results

If you attempt to interpret your lab results without knowing how to do so, you might really scare yourself. Although your medical provider is the expert, it helps to learn a little about the main aspects of your labs so you can watch your progress. These aspects include:

❏ **Absolute Neutrophil Count (ANC).** Measured in the CBC, neutrophils are a type of white blood cell (WBC). During treatment, you will notice that most of your white blood cells decrease, with the possible exception of basophils and eosinophils, which may increase. Although low neutrophils would be cause for alarm if you were on chemotherapy or had HIV, research shows that this reaction does not apply to patients undergoing HCV treatment. Standard practice, however, dictates that peginterferon be reduced if ANC drops to less than 750 cells/μL (cells per microliter) of blood. Medication is discontinued if ANC is less than 500 cells/μL. Some medical providers use drugs called *growth factors*, such as filgrastim (Neupogen), to stimulate white cell production in such cases. Growth factors are given by injection, have side effects, and are not for everyone.

❏ **Alanine Aminotransferase (ALT).** This liver enzyme is listed as part of the liver, or hepatic, panel. The normal range depends on the lab at which your blood work is performed. For instance, the normal range may be 5 to 40 IU/L (international units per liter) at one lab and 0 to 60 IU/L at another. Reference ranges also differ between men and women. Thankfully, labs list their own particular reference ranges on each report. ALT often increases when people drink alcohol or overload the liver with other toxic substances. Most patients have an elevated ALT before treatment begins. ALT often drops as treatment continues, but not always. A normal ALT during therapy is not a guarantee that the drugs are working, but it is a good sign that things are calming down in the liver. If ALT rises progressively or dramatically, the medication dose may be reduced or discontinued.

❏ **HCV Viral Load (HCV RNA).** It can be affirming to see your viral load steadily drop. The real thrill is when there is no sign of HCV, which is reflected on the lab report as "undetectable HCV RNA." As mentioned before, undetectable HCV by week four is an especially good indicator of treatment success, while detectable HCV at week twelve signals that the medication is not working.

❏ **Hemoglobin (HGB or HB).** Hemoglobin is the part of the red blood cell that carries oxygen to your cells. Your hemoglobin level is found in the CBC portion of the lab report. Ribavirin may cause the red blood cell to burst, which lowers hemoglobin and may result in a condition known as hemolytic anemia. This is a frequent occurrence and not generally cause for alarm. If your hemoglobin drops too low, however, it can be dangerous. For most patients, ribavirin doses are reduced if hemoglobin measures less than 10 g/dL (grams per deciliter), and stopped if less than 8.5 g/dL. Hemolytic anemia is a potentially serious condition, which is why close monitoring is essential. Patients with a history of cardiac disease may have their doses reduced at higher hemoglobin levels. This type of anemia has nothing to do with iron, so do not take iron supplements without medical supervision. Some medical providers will prescribe another medication, such as epoetin alpha (Epogen, Procrit), to stimulate red blood cell growth. It is given by self-injection, has some risks, and more research about its use for HCV is needed. Dehydration may also cause low hemoglobin, so it is important to drink sufficient water. Symptoms of low hemoglobin include fatigue, dizziness, and shortness of breath, much like being at high altitude. In fact, patients who spend time at high altitudes during their treatment may feel worse than when they are at sea level.

❏ **Platelets (PLT).** Platelets are responsible for blood clotting. Your platelet level is included in the CBC. Unlike hemoglobin, platelets can get quite low before there is cause for alarm. You actually won't feel the effects of low platelets, but you may see them. You may notice that it takes longer for your blood to clot or that you frequently have nose bleeds. If your level drops to less than 50,000 platelets/µL (platelets per microliter), the interferon dose is usually reduced. Interferon is usually discontinued if your level falls to less than 25,000 platelets/µL.

Store your health records in one place, whether it's a notebook, filing cabinet, computer, or box. If you store your information on a computer, though, make sure to keep a back-up copy. Other important records to keep include:

- contact information for all your medical providers

- emergency contact information

- health insurance information

- medical card or medical identification number

## CONDUCT YOUR RESEARCH CAREFULLY

I have a confession to make. Whenever I encounter a medical issue or receive a new drug from my doctor, I immediately look it up on the Internet. I rely on the Internet so much that if there were an Internet Anonymous group, I'd be a charter member. Despite my dependency on cyberspace, however, I must admit that its value is limited, as it is littered with misinformation. The trick is to find trustworthy sources.

If you are like me and find yourself searching the Internet more often than not, use the following tips to ensure that your research helps you rather than hinders you.

- **Avoid Self-Diagnosis.** After diagnosing myself with many diseases that never materialized, I made a point to break this habit. Leave the diagnoses to your medical provider.

- **Don't Panic.** If you read bad news about your condition online, don't panic. Yes, some people die from HCV, but the chances of this outcome are very low. Ease your mind by discussing your online investigations with your medical provider.

- **Don't Pay for Information.** Unless you are buying an article from a scholarly journal, never purchase research online. There is plenty of reliable free information on the Internet.

- **Know Your Source.** Government, educational, and non-profit websites are more likely to be unbiased than commercial websites. Commercial sites need to sell products and are more likely to feature information that supports this goal. Start your research with websites that end in .gov, .edu, or .org, rather than .com. Be cautious of any source that allows advertisements and does not mention anything about the person or organization behind it.

- **Look for Documentation.** Find research that includes the authors, medical affiliations, references, and dates. These facts can help you determine if the information is current and from a trustworthy source.

- **Narrow Your Search.** Use different search engines to narrow your investigation. For instance, *Google Scholar* is exclusively research-based and can be set to search only within recent publications. Additionally, *Yahoo Search* allows you to limit your search to .org, .gov, and .edu domains.

- **Protect Your Privacy.** Learn how to navigate the Internet safely. Do not provide personal information to any website, unless you trust it and know it is secure. Thankfully, most web browsers contain programs that help protect you from unsafe websites, and there are a number of antivirus software options on the market to safeguard your computer further.

- **Question What You Read.** Don't accept information found on websites as truth until you verify it. Be particularly skeptical of miracle cures.

- **Scrutinize Message Boards.** Don't be unduly influenced by stories you read on message boards or in discussion forums. These venues are great for tips and support, but personal experience and eye-witness accounts are not research.

Regardless of where you receive information, it helps to know how to interpret it. Reading medical literature is a skill that must be learned. The following points will teach you how to approach a medical study.

❑ **Be Critical.** As you read an article, ask questions. What is the point of the article? What is missing? What doesn't make sense?

❑ **Compare Oranges to Oranges.** If the subjects in a study were all Caucasian females over the age of forty, its results may not apply to a thirty-year-old Latino male. Don't assume all HCV patients are alike.

❑ **Keep an Open Mind.** We tend to look for facts that confirm our beliefs and ignore those that contradict our beliefs. An open mind is powerful because it can see the truth.

❑ **Consider Study Methods.** The gold standard in research is the *double-blind, randomized, placebo-controlled* study. This means that subjects are randomly assigned to groups, one of which receives a placebo (an inactive substance) while the other receives the actual medication being studied. No one, not even the research team, has any idea which group is taking the real drug. This type of research is much stronger than *observational* studies, which merely observe and report. Observational studies have value, but you shouldn't draw conclusions from them. Furthermore, *prospective* research, which hypothesizes an outcome and then records what happens over time, carries more weight than *retrospective* research, which draws conclusions from studies that have already occurred.

❑ **Stay Up-to-Date.** The HCV field is changing rapidly, so look for current research. It is best to find articles that were written in the past two years, but five to ten years may be acceptable, depending on the aspect of HCV being discussed.

❑ **Trust in Numbers.** Generally, studies that enroll lots of people (hundreds, thousands, or tens of thousands) carry more weight than small studies.

❏ **Trust Your Feelings.** Never let research, lab tests, or other people tell you how you feel. If the majority of HCV patients surveyed said they were depressed, this does not mean that you should or will feel depressed, too.

It is not enough to know the facts of a study; you need to know their significance and how they relate to you. Data are trivial without context. Always look at information and consider it in terms of your particular situation, because no one understands your illness as well as you.

## PREPARE FOR EMERGENCIES

Emergencies rarely happen during HCV treatment, but it is always wise to be prepared. In addition to 911, there are a handful of useful contacts to keep by your telephone or in your mobile phone's address book, including the telephone numbers of your health insurance company, medical provider, pharmacy, and hospital. Lastly, add your "in case of emergency" contact, or I.C.E., to your mobile phone and give that person a copy of your medical information. Lastly, since cell phone batteries die, keep a copy of your I.C.E. in your wallet.

Furthermore, everyone should have *advance directives*. This term refers to the legal documents that state your wishes for end-of-life care. I mention this important paperwork not because I want to frighten you or give you the false impression that you may die from treatment, but rather because it can be enormously helpful when this difficult time comes. Whether or not you are an HCV patient, be responsible and make this information available to your loved ones.

## ◼ THE BOTTOM LINE

Now that you've decided to undergo HCV treatment, the anxiety of failure may be overwhelming. The truth is that a little advance legwork and planning are all you need to increase your chance of success dramatically. The tips outlined in this chapter should put you on the right path and keep you there. Simply remember this advice:

❏ Before you begin HCV treatment, determine if you can afford it. If you cannot afford it, find out if you qualify for financial assistance or a clinical trial.

❏ Do not start treatment if you are breastfeeding, or if there is any possibility that you are pregnant.

❏ Prepare for your medical appointments by writing down and prioritizing your questions.

❏ Be organized and develop a system to remind you to take your drugs on time.

❏ Properly store all medication.

❏ Be aware that you will need regular labs and medical visits throughout treatment.

❏ Don't panic if you receive abnormal lab results. Some may be acceptable and even expected during HCV treatment. Your medical provider will let you know if there is cause for concern.

❏ Ask your medical provider for a list of conditions that constitute a medical emergency.

❏ Don't take dietary supplements except under medical supervision.

❏ Utilize the services that your drug manufacturer provides.

❏ Learn to use the Internet effectively. It can be a valuable resource.

❏ Keeping up with HCV research can provide valuable information, but you should never make decisions about your health based on an article or study. Go to your medical provider with questions.

❏ Find out if there are HCV support groups in your community.

Because the likelihood of beating HCV is so strong these days, I would hate for you to experience unsuccessful therapy due to a lack of diligence. You can reclaim your health by creating an environment that allows treatment to progress smoothly and effectively. Dedicate yourself to the process and you won't regret it.

# — 5 —

# HOW TO MANAGE
# THE SIDE EFFECTS OF
# HCV TREATMENT

*Extreme remedies are very appropriate
for extreme diseases.* —HIPPOCRATES

L ike the vast majority of HCV patients, you will probably
experience side effects during therapy, but you don't have to
suffer them helplessly. With proper management, side effects can be
eased or eliminated, thus improving your quality of life and treatment experience. In fact, effective side effect management is sometimes the critical ingredient that enables patients to finish HCV
therapy. And because a small problem is easier to fix than a big
problem, early intervention is one of the keys to successful treatment. This chapter details the physical and psychological side
effects most associated with HCV therapy and recommends techniques to alleviate them.

## PHYSICAL SIDE EFFECTS

HCV treatment can affect your body in many different ways. From
headaches and fatigue to gastrointestinal problems and insomnia,
the possible reactions to therapy are more than just a nuisance. It
seems that almost every part of the human body is vulnerable to the
side effects of HCV therapy. Your ears, nose, mouth, eyes, muscles,
skin, hair, and nails are all potential targets. But there are ways to
deal with these troubles, as you will soon discover.

## Flu-like Symptoms

Chills, fever, and body aches that feel like the flu are often an immune response triggered by interferon. These side effects are usually temporary, lasting four to six hours. Most people have mild flu-like symptoms after the first few injections or intermittently throughout treatment. If you are regularly in pain, talk to your doctor. Pain is symptomatic of many problems, and its cause needs to be determined. If you notice that these aches and pains regularly follow your interferon injection, ask your medical provider if it would be permissible to take a pain reliever before and, if necessary, after your shot. An over-the-counter option such as acetaminophen (Tylenol), aspirin, ibuprofen (Advil), or naproxen (Aleve) will usually take care of the problem. As a back-up plan, schedule your shot before bedtime in the hope that you might sleep through the worst of the reactions. Be sure to keep extra blankets and clothing next to your bed in case of severe chills, and take lukewarm sponge baths instead of hot showers if you are feverish.

## Headaches

Occasionally, you may get a dull headache. Describing his headache, one HCV patient said, "It feels like there is a headache coming on, but it never quite materializes." I think this statement captures the feeling perfectly. Minor headaches usually respond to over-the-counter pain relievers, such as acetaminophen, aspirin, ibuprofen, or naproxen. Limit the use of aspirin, ibuprofen, and naproxen, as overuse of these drugs may cause the headache to return once the relief wears off, also known as a *rebound headache*. If aspirin, naproxen, or ibuprofen works best for you, your medical provider might suggest ways to avoid rebound headaches, such as limiting use of the medication to twice a week or so, one day on, a few days off. If you are prone to headaches already, you may experience severe headaches or migraines, which should be evaluated by your doctor.

In addition to HCV medication, there are other factors that contribute to headaches, including sinus conditions and muscle tension. If you have a sinus headache, try steam inhalation, nasal lavage (irrigation), or self-massage to open your sinuses. Hot compresses applied to your sinuses may also provide relief. If the headache is caused by muscle tension or spasms, apply cold or hot compresses to the area that hurts most.

Dull headaches often respond to alternative medicine, such as acupressure. Try pinching the deep tissue between your thumb and forefinger with your other hand. Hold it for at least seven seconds and repeat until the headache fades. Aromatherapy may also be beneficial. Scents including lavender, peppermint, eucalyptus, and rosemary have been reported to soothe head pain. When I had a particularly stubborn headache, I would lie down in a dark room, cover my forehead and eyes with a small silk pillow filled with fresh lavender, and relax for a while. This worked better than pain relievers, so I recommend experimenting with essential oils applied to the temples, forehead, or base of the skull, or spraying your pillowcase with a favorite aroma. Scents, however, can also trigger headaches, asthma, or nausea, so stop this technique immediately if it doesn't help. Finally, staying adequately hydrated (see page 101) and practicing stress management (see page 111) may help you avoid headaches before they happen.

*Caffeine may cause or worsen a headache, but it can also lessen it. Keep track of your caffeine intake and see if it affects your headaches.*

## Muscle and Joint Aches

While HCV treatment typically causes intense but brief flu-like aches and pains that come soon after your injection, it also results in less severe but chronic muscle and joint aches, which require ongoing management. A hot bath may provide relief for aching muscles. Stretching and relaxing may also help, particularly if accompanied by soothing music. Massage, performed by you or a professional, can also be beneficial. In addition, visualization is a powerful pain management tool. If you doubt the power of mind over body, try the following exercise. Close your eyes and relax. Imagine someone handing you a big juicy lemon, and then feel yourself biting into it. Feel the juices running into your mouth and down your throat. Notice your reaction. If you felt a little tingle in your salivary glands, you just witnessed how visualization can affect the body.

To use visualization for pain management, find a comfortable position, close your eyes, and take a few deep breaths. Imagine that you are inhaling oxygen and sending it directly to your sorest spot. When you exhale, imagine that the pain is being carried out of your body. Do this for a while, relaxing with each breath. When you are ready to get up, stretch before resuming normal activities. Lastly, staying hydrated may alleviate this side effect, so drink plenty of water throughout the day.

## Eye Problems

During treatment, many patients experience dry eyes, and some complain about decreased visual acuity. Usually, these are minor, temporary problems that resolve themselves in time after therapy ends. In some cases, however, HCV medication causes permanent visual impairment if these side effects are ignored. If you already have an eye problem, HCV therapy could make the condition worse, so it is extremely important to have a routine baseline eye exam before beginning treatment.

Dry eyes may be soothed by a preservative-free lubricating solution. You may even need stronger reading glasses during treatment, but don't worry. You won't injure your eyes by increasing the magnification of your lenses, and if it is a temporary issue, you can return to a lower magnification later.

## Ear Problems

Although it is rare, hearing loss can occur during treatment, usually caused by thyroid problems that result from the medication. Your medical provider will check your thyroid levels regularly, but should you notice a problem hearing, report it immediately.

Some patients complain about dry, itchy ears. Never put anything smaller than your elbow in your ear, and avoid cotton swabs in particular. Swabbing your ears removes the wax, which contributes to itchiness. Cotton swabs can also damage your ears. If the itchiness is intense, try pressing the flap on the outside of each ear, as if you are blocking out noise. Try massaging around the ears a bit, or gently irrigate them with warm water.

## Nose Problems

Dry nasal passages can be itchy and painful. To alleviate this issue, use a saline nose spray to soothe the dryness, and then apply ointment such as Aquaphor, A and D ointment, or Vaseline just inside your nostrils. A humidifier may also help, especially if your house is dry. The nose is packed with tiny capillaries that break easily, so an itchy nose often leads to nosebleeds. If your platelets are low, it may be hard to stop the bleeding. When the nose bleeds, it looks like a massive amount of blood loss, which can be frightening, but it usually isn't as serious as it looks. To stop the bleeding, sit down, tilt your head slightly forward, and breathe through your mouth. If only one side is bleeding, press firmly on the outside of the nostril for ten minutes. If both sides are bleeding, pinch both nostrils shut for ten minutes.

If these methods don't solve the problem, continue to apply pressure for another ten minutes, for as long as thirty minutes. You may also apply ice wrapped in a towel or a bag of frozen peas to your nose. Once the bleeding has stopped, try not to blow your nose for twelve hours. If the bleeding hasn't ceased after thirty minutes, if the volume is such that you think you could fill a tampon in an hour or less, or if you feel weak or faint from blood loss, call your medical provider right away.

## Mouth Problems

Dry mouth is a common side effect of therapy and can lead to problems of the teeth and gums, and possibly infection. Staying hydrated and practicing good oral hygiene are strong preventative strategies. During my treatment, I picked up two good habits that

I still practice: daily flossing and brushing for two solid minutes. In addition, include tongue cleaning in your regimen. Some people use a brush to scrape the tongue, but a spoon is better. It is effective, causes less gagging, and can be sanitized in the dishwasher. If you notice bleeding gums, bad breath, or other dental problems, schedule an appointment with your dentist. I actually had my teeth cleaned every four months while I was on the medication. Here are some tips to help with dry mouth and bad breath:

- Sip water throughout the day.

- Ask your dentist or pharmacist for products specifically formulated to treat dry mouth.

- Chew on crisp fruits and vegetables, such as apples, jicamas, or carrots. The saliva production combined with the scouring action of the crisp foods is good for your teeth.

- Freshen your mouth by chewing a couple of seeds of anise, cardamom, coriander, or fennel. Chewing fresh parsley, mint, or sugar-free gum can also be beneficial.

Although less common, mouth sores affect some patients on HCV therapy. When sores are bad, it can be difficult to eat, and life can be miserable. For relief, avoid foods that are hard, crunchy, spicy, salty, or acidic. Do not drink liquids that are excessively hot. Ice or frozen juice bars may soothe mouth sores. Try over-the-counter products that numb canker sores or apply a protective barrier to the lesion. In addition, a used black tea bag placed on a mouth sore may also provide relief.

If mouth sores are bad and not alleviated by self-help measures, talk to your medical provider. There are a number of mouth sore solutions available by prescription. One is called *Magic Mouthwash*, which is a mixture generally used for cancer patients undergoing chemotherapy. One of its ingredients is viscous lidocaine, a liquid numbing agent. This mouthwash must be formulated by a pharmacist, but some pharmacists do not do formulations. Hospital, clinic-based, or independent pharmacies are your best bet in that case. Less effective but worth a try is a version that you can make yourself by mixing a teaspoonful of an antacid such as Milk of Magnesia (magnesium hydroxide) or Mylanta (aluminum and magnesium hydroxides) with a teaspoonful of liquid Benadryl (diphenhydramine). Swish it around your mouth for thirty seconds or so, and then spit or swallow four to six times daily.

Despite your best efforts, oral infections may still occur during HCV treatment, the most common being *thrush*. Thrush, also known as *candidiasis*, is a fungal infection that results from of an overgrowth of the mouth's normal bacteria, or *flora*. Antibiotics and stress may trigger this overgrowth. Signs of thrush include white cottage cheese-like lesions anywhere in the mouth, pain, and an odd taste in the mouth. If you take antibiotics, it is a good idea to take *probiotics*, which are healthful bacteria that your body needs. Yogurt with live or active cultures is a good source of probiotics. If you use inhalers, make sure you rinse your mouth after each use and keep your inhaler clean.

As you might expect, mouth dryness often causes chapped lips as well. Keep your lips well lubricated and avoid licking them, as doing so will cause them to dry out faster. Remove dead cells by rubbing your lips with a soft, dry washcloth or toothbrush. Moisten your lips by patting them with a soft, damp cloth, and then apply lip balm or lubricating jelly. A lip balm with sunscreen will protect your lips from sun damage.

*If your environment is dry, use a humidifier or cool air vaporizer to moisturize the air you breathe.*

## Skin Problems

Dry skin is so common during HCV treatment that I strongly advise patients to start moisturizing before the problem begins. Dry skin is itchy, and itching leads to scratching, which can get out of control and cause all sorts of problems, including irritated skin, sores, and infection. Rashes are another common side effect. Tell your medical provider as soon as you develop a rash, as they are much easier to treat in early stages. Another reason to report a rash immediately is that it could be a sign of an extremely rare condition called Stevens-Johnson syndrome, which is essentially a severe allergic reaction to a medication, infection, or illness. This syndrome begins with flu-like symptoms, but since these are also common side effects of HCV treatment, they are rarely given much thought. If, however, you develop a painful red or purplish rash that spreads quickly, report it right away. Blisters or swelling of the face, mouth, or tongue are other possible indications, as are hives and shedding of the skin.

You may notice that it takes longer for your skin to heal during HCV treatment. This is normal and partially due to dryness and other side effects of the medication. Swelling, pus, or pain, however, is not normal and requires medical attention. Your goal should be to prevent your skin from drying out, thus avoiding more serious consequences. Here are some basic tips to help with dry, itchy skin:

❏ Ask your medical provider about prescription or over-the-counter anti-itch medication, such as hydrocortisone cream.

❏ Don't use soap. Instead, use the moisturizing cleanser Cetaphil, or a similar product.

❏ Apply a fragrance-free hypoallergenic cream immediately after bathing. Cream is generally more effective than lotion. For extra protection, mix in a couple of drops of unscented lightweight body oil.

❏ For extreme dryness, rub A and D ointment or petroleum jelly between your hands and then apply a light layer over damp skin immediately after bathing.

❏ Drink a sufficient amount of water, as dehydration will dry out your skin.

❏ Try not to scratch. If you can't resist the urge, try rubbing itchy areas with an ice cube. If you scratch yourself in your sleep, wear cotton gloves to bed.

❏ Stay out of direct sunlight, wear protective clothing, carry an umbrella, and always use sunscreen. HCV medications can cause photosensitivity, which is a reaction to the sun that may cause you to itch, break out in hives, or burn more easily. If you do have a sun reaction, apply a cool compress of water or milk to the skin. Your medical provider may suggest an over-the-counter topical cortisone cream or prescribe something stronger.

❏ Avoid extremely hot showers and baths.

❏ Keep rooms ventilated and at a temperature of 60 to 70°F.

❏ Wear loose fitting clothes made from natural, breathable fabrics such as cotton or linen.

❏ Wash clothes and sheets with baby laundry soap or detergent formulated for sensitive skin.

❏ Use a humidifier in your room if you live in a dry climate or have central heating in your home.

Finally, an extremely common occurrence during therapy is redness at the injection site. It may be bright pink, deep red, or even slightly purple, and may remain colorful for a month or two. If there are red streaks or the area is warm, swollen, or oozing, alert your medical provider.

## Hair Problems

Patients worry about hair loss but usually find it to be minimal. Also, since it is gradual and scattered throughout the scalp, hair loss is barely noticeable to others. Significant loss of hair tends to occur more to men who are already prone to baldness. Nevertheless, you may worry until you see what happens. Do not expect to notice any hair loss in the first three months. I had a patient who ignored my assurances and shaved her head the day she started taking the medications. She spent the rest of her treatment watching her hair grow back.

You may have read warnings against using chemical preparations to color, perm, or process your hair during HCV therapy. Truly, the decision to use chemical hair products is an individual one based on your own circumstances, but let me assure you that taking HCV medications and using chemicals on your hair will not hurt your health. Granted, chemicals may damage your hair if it has already become dry from the HCV drugs, so it's best to choose the gentlest products possible with minimal chemicals. The main goal when doing your hair is not to heat it, as heat intensifies dryness. Employ the coolest setting on your blow dryer, and use curling irons sparingly. Even better, stop using blow dryers or switch to one made with the mineral tourmaline, which will dry your hair faster and with less heat. Here are other ways to maintain healthy hair.

❏ Shampoo your hair less often.

❏ Use dry shampoo instead of regular shampoo.

❏ Apply detangler or conditioner after you wash your hair.

❏ Brush your hair with a wide-toothed comb.

❏ Avoid devices that break the hair, such as clips, bands, or barrettes.

❏ Sleep on satin pillowcases.

You can also ask friends if they recommend any hair products that add body. If so, ask if you can sample a few before you make any purchases.

## Nail Problems

Brittle fingernails are an annoying side effect that you may be able to remedy or avoid by limiting the amount of time your hands are immersed in water, particularly hot water. Wear gloves when washing the dishes, preparing food, and gardening. Apply hand creams frequently, especially after you wash your hands, and use nail strengtheners. As always, be sure to stay hydrated.

*Drinking a sufficient amount of water is the single most important way to reduce skin, hair, and nail dryness.*

## Respiratory Problems

If you can't breathe, have chest pain, or are short of breath, call 911. If you have just walked, lifted something heavy, climbed stairs, or exerted yourself in any way, and your breathing improves after you stop the activity, you may have a fairly typical type of shortness of breath that occurs during HCV treatment. Since shortness of breath can be a symptom of medication-induced anemia as well as other more serious respiratory conditions, your provider ultimately needs to determine the cause of the problem. The same goes for chronic cough, which is generally not a big deal but may be a sign of something more serious. To combat a cough, drink plenty of liquids, suck on cough drops or sugarless lozenges, or try an over-the-counter cough medication. To soothe your mucous membranes, use steam or a humidifier and avoid irritants, such as smoke and cold air.

## Fatigue

Fatigue is a well-known and frustrating side effect of both HCV and its treatment. It leaves patients feeling mentally, spiritually, and physically handicapped. Exhaustion can cast a shadow on everything, hindering your capacity to perform the very tasks that may reenergize you. Just because it is a common side effect, however, doesn't mean that you have to live with it. Fatigue can be reduced, particularly if there is a clinical cause for it. HCV medications may cause thyroid abnormalities, anemia, depression, insomnia, and diabetes, each of which counts fatigue as a primary symptom, so it is critical to get a proper diagnosis before chalking it all up to a simple reaction to therapy. Your medical provider may prescribe drugs to help you, but you must be patient for results. Medication for depression or thyroid disorders may take two to six weeks to reach their maximum levels and be effective.

If there is no underlying clinical cause for your fatigue, other factors to consider are poor diet, dehydration, stress, and lack of exercise. If you aren't sufficiently hydrated, you may feel sluggish. The same is true for your diet. You don't expect your car to run without fuel or on low-quality gasoline, so why would you expect your body to run well without proper nourishment? (See Chapter 5 for more information on nutrition.)

If you are feeling stressed, try to let go of activities that are not totally necessary. HCV treatment is an important investment in your future, so weed out those tasks that are not serving your health. Prioritize your day, and set a pace that is reasonable for how you feel, rather than setting goals based on how much you used to do. Take shortcuts and ask for help. Ask friends to pick up groceries, make an occasional meal, or do some yard work. Plan to rest at regular intervals. Don't lay around thinking about how much you have to do or how terrible you feel. Instead, put on some music, watch the rain fall on the window, or listen to an inspiring audio book. Lastly, use humor, which is a remedy for both stress and fatigue. I have never been too tired to laugh. The Internet, movies, and television offer an endless supply of comic relief.

Although I resisted the concept for a long time, I must admit that positive affirmations can help lessen fatigue. I became convinced of this idea after I saw the results of research on chronic fatigue sufferers. In a study that divided chronic fatigue patients into two groups, one group was instructed not to do anything differently than they would normally, while the other group was asked to state the phrase, "I am getting my energy back" every time they felt tired. Those who repeated the positive affirmation reported significantly less fatigue.

Ultimately, physical activity is the best fatigue buster. During my therapy, keeping active helped me stay active. Once I stopped moving, it was hard to get going again, so my mantra was, "Just keep moving." In fact, physical fitness has a protective effect against the majority of side effects of HCV treatment in general, as you will see later in this chapter.

Finally, my last-resort remedy for fatigue is caffeine. During therapy, I sometimes drank four cups of green tea per day, stopping by the afternoon so the stimulant would not interfere with my sleep. Ask your medical provider if there is any medical reason why you should avoid caffeine. If there isn't, ask how much would be safe to consume in one day.

*I found ribavirin somewhat stimulating.*
*Since I required a total of five pills daily, I took*
*three of them in the morning and the other two*
*at 6:00 PM with an early dinner. If I took ribavirin*
*at bedtime, I tended to wake up in the middle*
*of the night, which led to daytime fatigue.*

## Insomnia

While HCV treatment makes you tired, the insomnia it can create just makes things worse. Losing a night's sleep is particularly problematic, as this influences how you function the next day. Sleep deprivation causes you to feel grouchy, which affects both your work and your personal relationships. Fortunately, insomnia is a side effect that is easily managed, and like all the other treatment side effects, the trick is to deal with it sooner rather than later.

The trouble with insomnia is that it is a huge problem at night, but in the light of day, we tell ourselves, "I am so tired that surely I'll sleep tonight." We don't call our medical providers because we hope the problem will go away. The longer we ignore insomnia, the more our bodies adapt to these new sleep cycles. I am not suggesting that you call your provider if you miss a night or two of sleep. If sleeplessness stretches into a week or two, though, you should get some help to determine its cause, as medical conditions such as overactive thyroid and depression can also promote sleep difficulties.

In addition to following the techniques mentioned in Chapter 3 (see page 50), you may want to try progressive muscle relaxation to beat insomnia. Start by contracting the muscles in your feet as tightly as you comfortably can. Keep them clenched for a few seconds, and then let go. Do the same with your calf muscles, tensing and relaxing. Continue moving up your body—thighs, buttocks, pelvis, and so on—up to and including your facial muscles. Relax all your muscles, from feet to head, and end by remaining quiet and breathing slowly. If you aren't allergic to it, add the smell of lavender to this routine, which may also help you drift off to sleep. Spray lavender scent on your sheet or pillow, apply lavender oil to your wrist or temple, or use a lavender-scented sachet inside your pillow or near your head.

If you wish to explore herbal supplements to treat your insomnia, never take anything without medical advice. Although valerian is a popular herb used to promote sleep, it is also known to be toxic to the liver. If you are considering an herbal blend that claims to improve sleep, make sure valerian is not an ingredient. A melatonin supplement may be helpful, but again, talk to your doctor before taking it.

If none of these tips get you to sleep, your physician may prescribe a sleep medication. Pharmaceuticals for sleep are much better than they used to be, and usually do not cause daytime drowsiness. If you are prone to substance abuse, however, tell your medical provider, as certain sleep medications are better than others for patients with dependency issues.

*Experts recommend getting seven to nine hours of sleep every night.*

## Lightheadedness

Occasionally, you may feel lightheaded or dizzy during HCV treatment. Report these symptoms to your medical provider so he can diagnose the specific cause. Therapy-related anemia and dehydration are two common reasons. If you feel dizzy or lightheaded, don't panic. Fear may intensify the problem, as it is common to hold your breath or breathe shallowly when scared. If you feel lightheaded, sit down and breathe deeply and slowly. If you feel faint, sit or lie down and tell someone that you feel faint. Drink some water and eat something if it has been a while since you last had food or liquids.

If you tend to feel lightheaded when you stand up, you may be able to prevent it by assisting your body's circulatory system. Before sitting or standing, pump blood to your upper body by squeezing the muscles in your legs and hips before and as you get up. Always stand up slowly.

*It does not seem logical to combat fatigue with exercise, but it really works. Take it easy and start small, but do it, especially when you don't feel like it.*

## Weakness

Some patients have bouts of weakness during treatment. This may be due to anemia, fatigue, or other side effects of HCV medication. Reduced activity may also be to blame. During my therapy, I didn't push myself at the gym, so naturally I lost muscle strength, which caused me to feel weaker. If you feel confused, or dizzy, are having trouble waking up, or are so weak that you can't get out of bed for over twenty-four hours, call your medical provider.

## Nausea and Vomiting

When I learned that nausea and vomiting are two of the side effects of HCV therapy, I was hesitant about starting the medications. As a nurse, I have never minded cleaning up vomit, but when it comes to my own stomach contents, I prefer they stay inside. As it turned out, I was nauseous quite often, so I personally researched many of the self-help and prescription treatments for the condition.

Ribavirin is the HCV drug typically responsible for creating stomach problems. Taking it with food may reduce stomach complaints. Hunger can intensify nausea, so eat a cracker or some other small piece of food every hour. Ginger helps with mild to moderate nausea. Try fresh ginger, crystallized ginger, or ginger tea. Some commercial brands of ginger ale are flavored with ginger, but technically there may not be sufficient ginger in them to be effective. Ginger ale, however, may still soothe the stomach, as might cola or other sodas. If carbonated beverages bother your stomach, let your soda get flat before drinking it. Peppermint, chamomile, or raspberry leaf tea may also alleviate the issue. If nausea is severe, your doctor may prescribe something for you or suggest an over-the-counter drug for relief, such as Pepto-Bismol, an antacid, or motion sickness medication. And since nausea is common during pregnancy, there are maternity-related products available, such as Preggie Pops or Queasy Drops, which help curb the feeling.

Finally, acupressure and acupuncture are effective tools to combat queasiness. Applying pressure to the inside of your wrist, approximately two finger widths above the crease where your hand meets your arm, is a helpful technique. Wristbands developed for motion sickness provide constant pressure on these points and are commonly sold in drugstores.

## Stomach Pain

Notify your medical provider if you have severe or chronic stomach pain. Mild stomach pain may be relieved by over-the-counter medications such as Pepto-Bismol, antacids such as Mylanta and Maalox, or some of the other methods mentioned in the previous section. Ask your medical provider which he recommends.

As stomach pain may be caused by hunger, try not to get too hungry. Eat small meals more frequently. If food bothers your stomach, try a clear liquid diet, including chicken broth, low-acid fruit juice, tea, and Jell-O. Rest after you eat, and avoid eating within a few hours of bedtime.

## Diarrhea

During HCV treatment, it is common to have loose or watery stools as a result of the medication. True diarrhea, such as the kind that keeps a person house-bound, is relatively uncommon. While it is not usually harmful, diarrhea can become dangerous or signal a more serious problem, so always see your medical provider if you have intense diarrhea that lasts for more than two days. If you have severe pain, fever, vomiting, black or bloody stools, or signs of dehydration such as intense thirst, dry mouth, dark urine, dizziness, and cold skin, report these conditions to your doctor immediately for evaluation.

Avoid both high-fiber and greasy foods if you have diarrhea. Your provider may recommend over-the-counter drugs such as Pepto-Bismol, Imodium, or Kaopectate. He may also suggest a bulk-forming laxative such as psyllium, which sounds counter-productive, but works on some types of diarrhea. Always remember that laxatives need to be taken with plenty of water.

Be sure to stay well hydrated and nourished. Drink small amounts of clear fluids frequently, as they are easier on the stomach. Consume liquids between meals rather than with your food. If you drink fruit juice, choose a brand without pulp. Fat-free chicken broth, tea with honey, and sports drinks are also good choices.

## Constipation and Hemorrhoids

Constipation is a frequent complaint during HCV treatment. It is usually due to dehydration, insufficient mobility, dietary changes, and changes in your normal schedule.

Regular bowel movements rely on adequate water, high fiber, and lots of activity. Drink lots of liquids, particularly warm or hot beverages in the morning. Fruit juices, particularly prune juice, may help. Exercise or simply walk regularly. Eat a high-fiber diet, including bran, prunes, and raw fruits and vegetables.

If you are constipated despite taking these steps, it may be time to consider over-the-counter assistance. Never take a laxative, though, if you have stomach pain, fever, or have been vomiting. Laxatives are intended for short-term use, not to exceed a week.

Start with something gentle such as polyethylene glycol 3350 (MiraLAX), psyllium (Metamucil), partially hydrolyzed guar gum (Benefiber), or methylcellulose (Citrucel). These may take a day or two to work and should be taken with plenty of water. If you still have a problem, ask your medical provider or pharmacist to recommend an effective over-the-counter laxative.

Constipation or hard stools may cause you to strain when you move your bowels, leading to swollen veins inside and around the anus, also known as *hemorrhoids*. According to clinical trials, this problem is more likely to affect patients that use telaprevir. Never postpone the urge to defecate out of fear of hemorrhoids, though, as doing so may make the constipation worse. You may notice a tinge of blood after you wipe yourself or feel itching, burning, or pain while defecating. Hemorrhoids usually calm down in a few days, assuming you find ways to solve the problem. Increasing your water and fiber intake should soften the stool and reduce the need to strain. If hemorrhoids remain, a gentle laxative, such as those already mentioned, may relieve discomfort incurred during bowel movements. Warm baths and over-the-counter hemorrhoid creams and ointments may also provide relief. If hemorrhoid pain is intense and does not go away after applying self-help measures, talk to your medical provider.

## Appetite and Taste Changes

Loss of appetite is a common side effect, but it does not occur in every case. If you are hoping that treatment will also serve as a weight-loss program, don't count on it. I have actually seen patients gain weight. It's true. One normally active patient gained quite a bit of weight during treatment because he thought that taking ribavirin with food meant he could eat huge bowls of ice cream topped with hot fudge on a constant basis. Between the extra calories and the reduced physical activity, he gained twenty pounds during therapy. Unwanted weight gain is distressing, particularly for those who experience other changes to their appearance due to the medication. As much as you can, eat healthful foods from the outset of treatment. Aim for a low-fat, high-fiber diet of colorful vegetables and hearty whole grains.

Rapid weight reduction, on the other hand, results in more than just lost fat; it can rob the body of muscle mass. Staying active, particularly by doing weight-bearing exercises, will prevent muscle loss. If you lose significant weight, be sure your medical provider monitors your medication, as some dosages may need to be adjusted accordingly. Anticoagulants, anti-diabetic agents, and drugs such as lithium, phenytoin, digoxin, theophylline, and valproic acid may reach toxic levels if enough weight is shed without a change in dosage. Weight-based doses of peginterferon and ribavirin may also need to be recalculated.

Some patients experience an odd or unpleasant taste in their mouth during therapy, often with a metallic flavor. Called *dysgeusia*, this phenomenon is common and usually not a cause for alarm. Clinical trials suggest that patients who take boceprevir during therapy may be more prone to this issue. Dental problems and certain medical conditions may also cause dysgeusia, though, so check with your medical provider and dentist, should it occur. To lessen the issue, try the following tips.

❑ Avoid metal, such as aluminum cans and canned products. Don't use metal cookware; cook with glass or crockery instead. Use plastic, wooden, or porcelain utensils when you eat.

❑ Before eating, rinse your mouth with club soda, warm salt water, or a mouthwash of half a teaspoon of salt, half a teaspoon of baking soda, and one cup of warm water.

❑ Drink sufficient water.

❑ Eat cold rather than hot foods, including sorbets, sherbets, frozen fruit bars, and smoothies.

❑ If a food does not taste good to you, take a holiday from it and try something new.

❑ If you normally take vitamin and mineral supplements that were not medically prescribed, stop taking them for a couple of weeks and see if your sense of taste returns to normal.

❑ Practice good oral hygiene.

❑ Season foods with aromatic herbs and spices. Try condiments such as horseradish or mustard, or tart flavorings, such as vinegar, lemon, lime, or orange. (Some people say that citrus and acid worsens the problem, so experiment with this idea.)

❑ Try sucking on sugarless hard candies.

Antidepressants such as citalopram may also affect taste. You should not, however, stop taking antidepressant medication without talking to your medical provider first, as doing so may cause serious consequences, including violent mood swings.

> *Changes in appetite and taste are temporary and should subside within two to twelve weeks of ending HCV therapy.*

## Menstrual Irregularities

There is not much information regarding HCV treatment's effect on the menstrual cycle, but women have noticed irregularities while undergoing therapy, reporting changes in their menstrual flow and cycle length. Some women report less premenstrual syndrome (PMS) symptoms, while others report more. It is likely that your menstrual cycle will return to its pre-treatment regularity once therapy ends, unless you are nearing menopause, in which case, it may not.

## Sexual Changes

Sexual side effects of HCV treatment include vaginal dryness, diminished sexual desire, sexual dissatisfaction, erectile dysfunction, and problems with ejaculation. These issues typically begin a month into treatment and resolve within six months of ending therapy. Sexual intercourse may be uncomfortable, even painful, due to vaginal dryness. Lubricants can relieve this problem, but do not use petroleum or oil-based products, particularly if using barrier contraception, as oil can destroy condoms and diaphragms.

Although HCV medications can directly affect sexual function, there may also be other factors at play. If you feel tired or unwell, you may not be interested in sex. If your hair and skin have lost their luster, you may not feel attractive, which may dampen your libido. Some antidepressant medications may also interfere with sexual function. To identify the main cause, consult your physician. You may feel uncomfortable about the matter, but let me reassure you that it is a common conversation between patients and providers. Former Senator Bob Dole may have lost his bid for the presidency, but he changed the country by openly discussing his erectile dysfunction. His bravery made it possible for many others to talk about the issue.

Drugs such as tadalafil (Cialis), sildenafil (Viagra), and vardenafil (Levitra) may help erectile dysfunction. Ask your doctor if these are safe and appropriate for you. If so, request free samples or look for money-saving coupons on the Internet. If antidepressants are contributing to your sex problems, your provider may recommend a different medication or suggest a way of taking antidepressants that may relieve the issue. But remember never to change or stop your antidepressant dose without your doctor's approval and supervision.

The most damaging aspect of this side effect is the consequence it can have on your relationship with your partner. Your partner may feel rejected, so make it clear that the problem is a temporary medical setback. Open and honest communication helps. Find ways that you can still share intimacy, such as a candlelit dinner, holding hands at the movies, or giving each other a massage.

## RELIEF OF PHYSICAL SIDE EFFECTS

While each of the recently outlined physical side effects of HCV treatment may be alleviated or managed in its own particular way, there are a few lifestyle habits that you can adopt to help generally ward off the worst of these reactions. As you may have noticed in the previous section, hydration plays a role in lessening many of the side effects of therapy. On top of that, nutrition and physical fitness can also facilitate the achievement of a smooth treatment program. When it comes to maintaining your health, these simple ideas are just as valid today as they were in the past, and as they are sure to remain in the future.

### Hydration

While drinking a sufficient amount of water is important for overall health, it is even more so for people undergoing HCV treatment, as dehydration makes the side effects of HCV drugs more intense. Patients report more fatigue, headaches, and joint pain during therapy when they are not properly hydrated. Signs of dehydration include intense thirst, severe dry mouth, dark urine, dizziness, and pale cold skin. When it comes to the right amount of liquid to drink, however, it seems no one is really sure how much it might be. There are weight-based suggestions, gender guidelines, and calculations based upon the amount of liquid lost throughout the day, but nothing definitive. I suggest you drink eight ounces of liquid, eight times a day, and then look at the color of your urine. If it is medium or dark yellow, drink a little more. If it is pale yellow, you are probably consuming the right amount. If your urine is clear, you could cut back.

While water is the best liquid to drink for hydration, it can get boring. You can flavor your water by adding slices of fresh orange, lime, lemon, ginger, cucumber, or sprigs of mint. Hot water with honey, lemon, or mint is another alternative. If you get tired of water, there is always the option of tea. Herbal teas may even soothe an upset stomach, clear congestion, or help with a headache. If you don't like water, hot or cold, there are other choices, such as juice or soda, though these are not the best choices due to their high sugar content. Although diet beverages do not contain sugar, they do contain many other artificial ingredients, so again, water is a better choice. As a compromise, you could always mix commercial beverages such as lemonade, soda, or fruit juice with club soda or sparkling water, thereby reducing both the content of questionable additives as well as your costs.

It is recommended that you drink water before you are thirsty, sipping it throughout the day instead of gulping it. To help you remember to drink, keep water in places you frequent, such as your favorite chair at home, where you work, or in the car. You can also trick yourself into drinking more water by using short, wide beverage glasses, rather than tall, skinny ones.

*If you or your partner can become pregnant, remember to use two effective forms of birth control, such as a condom and spermicidal jelly.*

## Nutrition

Nutrition directly affects your ability to function. Never skip a meal, even if you don't feel like eating. Eat small portions every three to five hours. If you have no appetite, entice your taste buds by offering them variety. Try foods of different textures, tastes, and temperatures, such as warm soup, cool smoothies, or savory snacks. In addition, give the foods you've never liked another shot. Some people acquire a taste for dishes they once hated. Do your best to choose items that have high nutritional value, and be sure to eat a sufficient amount of protein each day. Fish, poultry, or lean red meat (twenty-one grams of protein per three-ounce piece), yogurt (eleven grams of protein per cup), eggs (seven grams of protein per egg), beans (sixteen grams of protein per cup), and peanut butter (nine grams of protein per two tablespoons) are all good options. Adult women need about forty-six grams of protein every day, while men need about fifty-six grams.

Food that is fresh and whole is better for your health than processed food. Unfortunately, as your appetite declines, so does your energy level. As a result, you may not want to shop for food or prepare it. Do yourself a favor and put together extra meals while you have the energy to do so and store them in the freezer. Also, opt for meals that don't involve a lot of preparation, such as a vegetable omelet, low-salt tortillas chips with bean dip, or last night's leftovers. Finally, keep nutritious snacks on hand, including applesauce, trail mix, and sliced fruit. Although they do not fit into the category of fresh and whole, nutritional drinks such as powdered instant breakfasts, Ensure, or similar products from your local health food store may also be helpful when you truly lack the strength to eat optimally.

## Physical Fitness

Staying active is one of the best methods of managing the side effects of HCV therapy. Interferon can lead to aches, pains, and stiffness, which are made worse by immobility. In fact, inactivity can create or worsen all sorts of problems, including fatigue, depression, insomnia, and constipation. It can also result in low bone density, known as *osteopenia*, as well as severe loss of bone density, known as *osteoporosis*.

If you think you won't be able to engage in physical fitness during therapy, think again. Some patients actually accomplish amazing feats. One patient I know climbed a 14,000-foot mountain, while another bicycled 200 miles every week. One patient skied all winter, while another never missed his regular gym workout. Of course, most people won't be quite so active, but the facts are inspiring. I managed to walk every day during treatment, although I was so slow by the end that my dog began to give me dirty looks.

Walking, swimming, stretching, yoga, Pilates, Tai Chi, and Qi Gong are excellent ways to remain active, flexible, and in good shape. Choose an activity and look for classes in your community or online, or check out a book on the subject at your local library. To prevent bone loss, engage in weight-bearing exercises, and be sure to get adequate calcium and vitamin D. The sun is the best source of vitamin D, but with the danger of skin cancer and the photosensitivity caused by HCV medication, supplements are often the best way to insure adequate doses. Your medical provider can advise you about the right dosages for your age and situation.

You don't have to dedicate a great deal of time to staying fit. In fact, while you are on treatment, it is better to limit exercise to brief periods. Aim for a total of thirty minutes daily, or slightly longer if you are accustomed to physical activity. You can break the time up into intervals of five, ten, or fifteen minutes. For strength training, use light weights or exercise bands. If you don't own hand weights, water bottles or cans of soup are good substitutes. Finally, try to incorporate physical fitness into your normal, everyday routine. Park the car at the far end of the parking lot, take the stairs, vacuum, or do some gardening. A walking buddy makes time pass more quickly, so go for a stroll with a friend. Stretch or lift weights while watching your favorite television show.

## Complementary and Alternative Medicine

Complementary and Alternative Medicine (CAM) involves more than just dietary supplements; it includes healing practices from all over the world. Some CAM practices use combinations of herbs, nutrition, bodywork, and lifestyle changes. *Naturopathy*, which promotes the use of the human body's "vital energy" as a means of overcoming illness; *Ayurveda*, which finds the basis of healing in the five elements of the universe (earth, water, fire, air, and ether); and traditional Chinese medicine are but a few examples. Some western medical practitioners are supportive of CAM, while others are not. But the reverse is also true. Many CAM practitioners believe only in their own techniques. If you have done your research and decide that a particular course of action is right for you, be sure to remain cautious and knowledgeable of it. New information on various health practices is always surfacing. If any alternative therapies interest you, be sure to tell your traditional medical provider that you will be seeing a CAM practitioner, and always let your CAM practitioner know that you have HCV. Never withhold information from the people who are trying to help you.

*Set reasonable, achievable exercise goals and keep them flexible. Some days you may need to do less. Always do something, though, as staying active is important.*

Just to be on the safe side, I personally endorse only those healing arts that don't pose any risk to the liver or involve taking herbs. If you choose, however, to use a form of CAM that includes herbs, see the full discussion of supplements on pages 42 to 47. I appreciate alternative practices such as acupuncture, acupressure, massage, Tai Chi, and meditation, which don't require ingesting supplements or any other possibly problematic substances. Furthermore, there is valid research that proves the effectiveness of these methods against pain and nausea. Some insurance companies even offer discounts on these types of CAM. If you don't have health insurance, see if there is a school of Chinese medicine in your community that has a low-cost clinic. One advantage of acupressure is that you can perform it on yourself once you have had a few sessions and are familiar with the process. There are also many online resources that can teach you how to use it effectively. (See the Resources on page 148.)

Herbal teas, spices, and certain foods may also help with mild HCV treatment side effects. Ginger, chamomile tea, raspberry leaf tea and peppermint tea may alleviate nausea and digestive distress. Chicken soup or chamomile tea may help relieve dry or stuffy mucous membranes. If you decide to try these methods, choose brands from reputable sources, and avoid imports from unfamiliar sources where product contamination might be a risk. Remember, herbs have the power to help, but they also have the power to harm. Use common sense before you take anything, and always clear it with your doctor first.

## PSYCHOLOGICAL SIDE EFFECTS

In addition to causing physical side effects, HCV medications can affect brain chemistry, resulting in psychological conditions, including depression, anxiety, and anger, about which you will learn in the following section. A certain amount of this side effect is normal, but extreme changes in mood are an entirely different matter. Thoughts of hurting yourself or others, severe depression or anxiety, and rage are serious issues that require immediate help. If you have these thoughts, call your medical provider or 911 right away.

### Depression

If you have never been depressed, you may be surprised to learn that sadness is not its only symptom. According to the National Institute of Mental Health, depression can include:

- crying spells without a reasonable explanation

- difficulty concentrating, sometimes accompanied by memory problems and an inability to make decisions

- fatigue, insomnia, or other sleep-related problems

- feeling anxious or "empty" on a regular basis

- guilt, worthlessness, or helplessness

- hopelessness or pessimism

- irritability

- loss of interest or enjoyment in hobbies, social activities, and sex

- overeating and weight gain, or loss of appetite and weight loss

- thoughts of death or suicide, or suicide attempts

Patients experience depression in different ways. Men are more likely to notice irritability, insomnia, and loss of interest in activities, while women will more often express feelings of sadness, guilt, or worthlessness. Antidepressants can be a tremendous help with this psychological side effect of HCV treatment. Your provider can recommend the appropriate one for you. If you take an antidepressant but still feel depressed, you may need a dose adjustment or an additional medication to augment the one you are taking. If you have insomnia along with depression, it may be best to take a drug that also acts as a sedative. If fatigue is a problem, then perhaps a stimulating antidepressant would be better for your situation. Keep in mind, though, that these medications can take from two to eight weeks to work, and that you may need to try several antidepressants before finding the one that suits your needs.

If you take antidepressants during therapy, your physician will likely ask you to remain on them for a few months after HCV treatment ends, tapering your dosage until you can stop safely. I have known too many patients who stopped taking their antidepressants the moment their HCV therapy concluded, and with distressing results, including flu-like symptoms, headache, nausea, and intense psychological reactions, some of which lasted for weeks or longer.

If you would like to try using a dietary supplement against depression instead of a pharmaceutical, proceed with caution. Although research shows that St. John's wort may be an effective treatment for mild to moderate depression, there is no evidence to suggest it would be useful against depression related to HCV therapy. In fact, St. John's wort is prohibited if you are taking telaprevir or boceprevir. Because supplements may negatively interact with HCV medications, it is highly recommended that you speak to your medical provider before taking any substance along with HCV drugs.

## Anxiety

I battled anxiety while on treatment. It was quite uncomfortable, especially since the more I noticed my anxious feelings, the worse they got. Fortunately, I recognized that my anxiety cropped up a couple of hours after I took the ribavirin. Identifying this pattern helped tremendously, as I was able to tell myself that it would pass. All I had to do was focus on something else. I was still anxious, but I wasn't anxious about *being* anxious.

More intense than this feeling but certainly less common is mania. Although HCV treatment may induce mania, it is more likely to show up when people start taking antidepressant medications. The symptoms of mania include:

❏ Decreased need for sleep

❏ Excessive talking

❏ Feeling overly excited without a reasonable explanation

❏ Inappropriate social behavior

❏ Increased sexual desire

❏ Irritability

❏ Markedly increased energy

❏ Poor judgment

❏ Racing thoughts

If you experience any of these side effects, make an appointment with your doctor.

## Anger and Rage

Some patients, particularly men, report feelings of anger and rage while taking HCV medication. Anger is an emotion; rage is anger that is out-of-control, and often occurs when anger is not dealt with appropriately. These side effects may cause a great deal of problems, especially at home and in the workplace.

If you have feelings of anger or rage, your doctor may prescribe an antidepressant. Anger management techniques, which can be learned by attending an anger management group or researching online, are also good ways to cope with such damaging emotions. (See the Resources on page 148.)

## RELIEF OF PSYCHOLOGICAL SIDE EFFECTS

While the physical side effects of HCV treatment can be tough, the psychological reactions to therapy can be just as debilitating, and many times more difficult to manage. Dry skin can be alleviated through simple means such as proper hydration, but mood-related issues such as anger and stress must be addressed a little more abstractly. Maintaining a positive attitude, letting go of stress, and finding humor in life are all hard feats to accomplish, but they are not impossible. If you change your mindset, you will transform the way you experience HCV therapy.

### Managing Your Mood

Knowing that HCV treatment affects brain chemistry, I once thought that telling HCV patients to stay positive was about as useful as telling someone to smile during a root canal. Despite this belief, I actually learned that a good attitude makes the unbearable become bearable. I was not a naturally positive person, but I became one by watching other HCV patients.

The patient from whom I learned the most was a woman in her sixties with cirrhosis. In the middle of HCV treatment, her husband died unexpectedly. He was her sole support, and because of some estate issues, she lost her house and medical insurance. She had been quite sick even before treatment, yet she did not quit HCV therapy. The amazing thing was that she had initially been very frightened and resistant to the idea of HCV treatment. She was so fearful that I didn't think she was going to try it. Throughout treatment, however, she became an inspiration to me. She said, "When you have nothing left to lose, life is easier to live. You know you can survive even after you have lost everything." So when the going got tough during my own therapy, I thought of her.

Learning to control your attitude makes a huge difference in the way you experience HCV therapy. Often, you can talk yourself out of a mood. If you notice negative thoughts bobbing about in your head, counteract them with positive thoughts. You may need to do this repeatedly all day, and it isn't always the most simple thing to do, but the ability to transform negative thoughts into positive ones gets easier with practice. One trick is to look for opportunities, not problems. If getting out of bed is hard, then perhaps it's a good time to talk to a friend over the phone. If you feel too sick to go to work, see it as an opportunity to stay at home and watch the birds outside your window. There is always a brighter side to life if we just look for it. Here are some other tips to help you manage your moods effectively:

❑ Be on guard for negative thoughts. Replace negative messages with positive ones. If you tell yourself you can't make it another day, remember that you've made it through hard days before and will make it through more.

❑ Call someone else who may be struggling or in pain.

❑ Don't feel sorry for yourself. It's normal to do so, but it doesn't help anything. Say, "I don't *have* to undergo treatment, I *get* to undergo treatment" and see if that changes your mood.

❑ Focus on what is working rather than what isn't.

❑ Identify what you have control over and what you don't. For instance, you can't control other people, but you can regulate how much time you spend with people who irritate you.

❑ Make a list of everything you have to be grateful for, including the opportunity to receive HCV treatment.

❑ Make sure you get enough sleep every night.

❑ Perform some type of physical activity on a daily basis. Keep moving, even if you don't feel like it, as exercise can revitalize and restore your positive outlook.

❑ Remember that you are on a journey and what you are feeling is temporary.

❑ Start with acceptance. You may *want* a better attitude, but you have the one you have. You can't change your mindset until you accept yourself. Don't be too hard on yourself, but don't stop trying to improve yourself.

Finally, use visualization to help defeat negativity. Picture your thoughts as birds flying through your head. If negative thoughts spend too much time there, imagine them flying away. Invite positive thoughts to build nests in your head. If negative thoughts won't go away, write down what is bothering you on a piece of paper and put it in a box. Take the paper out of the box once a day and think about it for a brief period of time, perhaps twenty minutes, and then put it back in the box. If the thoughts come back, remind yourself that they are in the box, and you can think about them later.

## Beating Stress

HCV treatment makes it difficult for you to keep up with your normal activities, which may cause you to feel overwhelmed and stressed. Personally, when my car ran out of gas during my time on HCV drugs, I didn't know which to call first, a tow truck or a crisis hotline. Because it is hard to remain positive while under stress, it is a good idea to learn strategies to manage this emotion. Perhaps the best way to do so is to simplify your life. Don't put so much pressure on yourself. Prioritize your needs and lower your expectations. Write a to-do list of the most important things you have to do and don't fret about the minor issues. Additionally, learn to say no. You will feel a heavy weight lifted off your shoulders when you do.

As mentioned in Chapter 3, learning how to meditate can also help, especially if practiced regularly. (See page 54.) Stress and worry cause the muscles to tense up, robbing the body of valuable energy. By understanding how to relax, you will find residual power to help you get through the rest of the day. If meditation doesn't interest you, try an activity that offers similar benefits. Nature walks, attending a baseball game, birdwatching, golfing, and listening to music can all be calming.

> *When times get tough, try saying,*
> *"This too shall pass."*

## Finding Humor

Above all, keep a sense of humor. Laughter can sustain you through pain. As Mark Twain said, "Humor is mankind's greatest blessing." Whether you're reading the paper, watching television, or going to the movies, choose comedic fare rather than dark topics. Put joke books in your bathroom and by your bed for those extra minutes you find throughout the day. The healing properties of laughter are backed by solid scientific research. When you laugh, your body experiences a cascade of healthy chemicals, boosting your immune system, brain, hormones, and so on. At the very least, humor certainly helped me deal with my temper while I was on HCV medication.

If you really want to laugh, join an HCV support group. No one understands how poorly you feel better than a fellow patient who has experienced treatment. I can't explain why humans find humor in shared misery, but we do, and it helps.

## WHEN TO CALL YOUR DOCTOR

While this chapter outlines the average physical and psychological side effects of HCV treatment, along with ways in which you might handle them, the following side effects require urgent attention. Before starting treatment, review this list with your medical provider to see if he would make any changes to it. Call your doctor immediately if you experience any of the following conditions:

❑ bloody diarrhea

❑ blurred, decreased, or loss of vision

❑ chest pain

❑ difficulty breathing beyond the shortness of breath that comes with exertion

❑ excessive fatigue or weakness that prevents you from getting out of bed

❑ hearing loss

❑ persistent fever over 100°F, or one that continues to elevate

❑ rash with fever, blisters, or sores in the mouth, nose, or eyes

❑ red or inflamed eyes

❑ severe pain in your stomach or lower back

❑ swelling of the face

❑ unusual bleeding or bruising

❑ weakness, loss of coordination, numbness, or difficulty speaking

*Hand washing is your best protection against unwanted illnesses. Wash your hands for twenty to thirty seconds—about the time it takes to sing the alphabet song slowly.*

## THE BOTTOM LINE

The key to managing the possible side effects of HCV treatment successfully is to deal with them before they become bigger problems. Whether it is a physical reaction or a psychological one, there are methods you can learn to alleviate it considerably. Sometimes the answer to lessening a side effect is as simple as drinking more water, sometimes you may need an over-the-counter pharmaceutical, but in most cases, help can be found. You just need the right information. So remember, never worry about bothering your medical provider with your questions; that is part of his job. Now that you are undergoing treatment and likely experiencing some of the reactions to the medication, here are a few points to keep in mind:

❏ Many side effects can be avoided or minimized by staying hydrated and physically active.

❏ Don't be afraid to take medication for aches and pains if you are able to do so safely. There is no reason to suffer.

❏ No research has been done on the use of herbs and supplements during HCV treatment. Use supplements with caution, and inform your medical provider about any substance you wish to take.

❏ If you are having trouble breathing, seek immediate medical attention.

❏ Food is fuel. Eat small frequent meals, and choose a nutritious diet.

❏ Take precautions to avoid pregnancy.

❏ It's hard to function when you are sleep deprived. Tell your provider if you are having sleep difficulties.

❏ Changes in mood are common side effects that are best helped by early intervention.

❏ Learn how to manage stress, and keep life simple.

❏ Join an HCV support group. Patients who have experience with HCV treatment often have good tips on how to handle side effects.

Above all else, nurture and indulge your sense of humor. Some day you may look back at this and laugh, so why wait? Laughter will do you more good than you realize, so laugh now when you need it.

# — 6 —

# HOW TO MANAGE YOUR LIFE WHILE UNDERGOING HCV TREATMENT

*Isn't everyone a part of everyone else?* —BUDD SCHULBERG

The physical and psychological side effects caused by HCV medications aren't relegated to you alone. They often spill over into your work life, your personal life, and your sex life, affecting the people around you. With all the ups and downs of therapy, as well as the time spent focusing on yourself throughout the drug program, you may not know what to do about everyone else. This chapter outlines the private and public difficulties that you may face in the major aspects of your life as a result of HCV treatment and details ways in which you can successfully deal with these troubles. It's not an easy road, but it is one you can handle, and one that you do not have to travel alone.

## WORK LIFE

Because work is a significant part of life, most HCV patients understandably wonder if treatment will negatively affect their productivity and relationships at the workplace, or worse, if they will have to take medical leave during therapy. Since HCV medication can affect different people in different ways, it is impossible to predict how you will function in the work environment. The majority of patients I have known, however, were able to manage well enough

115

to work satisfactorily throughout treatment. In fact, work often provided them with a focus other than therapy, distracting them from side effects, making them feel useful, and helping them successfully complete the regimen.

On the other hand, your job may be so physically or emotionally demanding that it interferes with your ability to finish treatment. If this is the case, you may need to disclose your condition and talk to your supervisor about modifying your responsibilities or workload. If your job involves hard physical labor, you may need to request lighter duties. Other possible job-related circumstances, including working at an elevated height, being exposed to the sun, or handling chemicals, should also be modified. Finally, if you have a high-risk occupation, such as smokejumping or race car driving, let your medical provider know before you begin therapy. Such stressful jobs may not be compatible with treatment.

> *Keep your life simple. Try not to take on too much outside of work. Delegate tasks to others, prioritize, take shortcuts whenever possible, ask for help, and lower your standards. You don't have to do everything perfectly.*

It generally isn't necessary to decide whether or not to work during therapy until you learn how HCV drugs affect you. It may be possible to continue working by taking occasional sick days, reducing your total hours or days on the job, or modifying your responsibilities. But even if treatment may seem like a breeze at the beginning, be careful not to act as though nothing has changed. I functioned poorly at work when I pushed as I had in the past, ignoring my body's signals, neglecting to take breaks, and opting to eat lunch at my desk. Although I resisted advice to take it easy at first, eventually I saw that I was more efficient when I took breaks periodically. I liked to stretch my legs and clear my head by taking a walk outdoors, where the scenery and fresh air always perked me up. In the afternoon, I either put my head down on my desk or reclined in my car for a short nap. I believe these brief interludes were the reason that I was able to work throughout treatment.

## Disclosure

Most likely, you'd rather not say anything about your HCV. Although you have a right to keep your condition private, maintaining that privacy can get tricky during treatment when others notice that you aren't quite yourself. If the quality of your work slips or your coworkers begin inquiring about your well-being, it may be better to admit that you are on medication that has a number of side effects, without going into specifics. Being too vague, however, could result in an awkward work atmosphere, so you may ultimately decide to disclose your condition.

Disclosing your HCV at the workplace can be difficult, particularly if you work with children or seniors, in the healthcare field, or in food services. The reality is that there are safety protocols for occupations that involve working with the public, and when these standards are observed, the risk of infecting others with HCV is virtually eliminated. Unfortunately, your coworkers and the general public may not understand this fact. *You* may know that you aren't putting other people at risk, but convincing other people is an entirely different matter. Moreover, there is a stigma associated with HCV, partly because it is an infectious condition, and partly because it is often linked to intravenous drug use, whether drug use was the source of infection or not. I have even heard HCV sufferers stigmatize other HCV patients. I cringe when I hear a patient talk about being "innocently" infected by a blood transfusion. This word implies that anyone who gets HCV from drug use is guilty and somehow deserves the virus. HCV patients who catch the disease through drug use don't need the extra guilt. They tend to beat themselves up incessantly for having engaged in a behavior that led to infection. None of these attitudes is productive or helpful.

To shake the stigma, begin by examining your own attitude towards HCV. You have the opportunity to heal more than just this disease; you can heal your mind and spirit too. You don't require medication to cure your guilt and shame. All you need to do is let go of these useless emotions. Once you do, you will experience a freedom that promotes deeper healing than you thought possible. Personally, I have always been open about having HCV; but, I must admit, my honesty has not always been met with good results. Over the years, some people have acted as if the virus was going to leap out of my body and infect them. In fact, my babysitter quit after her parents heard that I had HCV. Most people, however, are simply curious about the disease, and I welcome the opportunity to inform them on the subject. Disclosing your HCV is an undoubtedly hard and personal decision to make, but the truth is that hiding in shame may be just as difficult.

> *You don't have to accept the stigma associated with HCV. As Eleanor Roosevelt said, "No one can make you feel inferior without your consent."*

## Risk of Occupational Transmission

While most people consider the healthcare profession the riskiest job in terms of HCV transmission, there are many other jobs that pose a similar danger. Firefighters, police officers, military personnel, athletes, janitors, house cleaners, and cosmeticians may come into contact with blood while at work. If you have HCV and work in a field where there is the potential for blood-to-blood contact, you should be adequately trained to prevent disease transmission. Training is for your safety as well as the safety of others. If you have not received instructions on how to avoid disease transmission, discuss the matter with your employer.

The healthcare field follows a system of strict rules known as *universal precautions* in order to reduce the risk of disease transmission. The effectiveness of these precautions is demonstrated by the fact that the rate of infection of healthcare workers is close to that of the general population. If you are in the cosmetics or personal care industry, however, you may not have adequate access to safety information, particularly if you are self-employed. In most states, jobs such as manicurist, esthetician, barber, and hair stylist are licensed professions, so you can check your state's licensing agency for guidelines.

## Job Protection and Disability Benefits

The Americans with Disabilities Act (ADA) regulates what your potential employer can and cannot ask you. You are not required to disclose that you have HCV or that you are undergoing treatment, but you may be asked if your health will limit your ability to perform the job adequately. While you must answer the question truthfully, you do not have to reveal any specifics or even speculate about future performance levels. If you know you have HCV and may one day undergo treatment, but your current condition is such that it will not affect your work, it is unnecessary to divulge any health-related information. If, on the other hand, you are already taking HCV medication and not feeling well, you must be honest about your limitations, though you need not disclose the exact cause of the problem. The ADA's protection, however, does not cover everyone. It applies only to private employers, labor unions, employment agencies, and state and local governments that have fifteen or more employees. (Federal government employees have similar coverage under the United States Equal Opportunity Commission.)

Keep in mind that you are safeguarded under the ADA only if your employer is aware that you have a medical condition that can affect job performance. For instance, the ADA may protect you if you tell your boss that you to need a thirty-minute break every afternoon due to fatigue from treatment. Your employer may not grant your specific request, but she must make reasonable accommodations. If you don't tell your employer about your medical problem, you will have no protection if you decide to take a quick nap every day at your desk and get fired as a result. If you need to adjust your work routine in order to do your job, your medical provider can write a letter to your employer's Human Resources office.

It is also important to know that the ADA protects you only during the hiring process and while you are actually working. It does not protect you if you are no longer able to work. While the ADA will help you continue to work, if you cannot perform the essential duties of your job, you may be let go. In addition, if you've applied for and received a job offer, you may be asked to take a physical. If the exam casts doubt on your potential to perform the job satisfactorily, the offer of employment may be legally withdrawn, assuming no reasonable accommodations can be made to assist you in meeting the fundamental requirements of the job.

If your work cannot be modified and you must take time off, look into your company's short-term and long-term benefits. You may also qualify for time off under the Family and Medical Leave Act (FMLA). If you are unable to work and your place of employment qualifies, you may be able to take up to twelve weeks of unpaid leave under the FMLA.

## PERSONAL LIFE

As an HCV patient, the virus touches more than just you; it also affects your family and friends. This is most apparent during treatment when you are vulnerable and not quite yourself. One of my lowest moments occurred during HCV therapy. I had a huge temper tantrum over an insignificant issue. I yelled at the two most important people in my life, my husband and daughter, claiming they were insensitive. Just before slamming the door to my bedroom, I shouted, "This is your fault and has nothing to do with the medication!" A year later, when I was back to being my gentler, more compassionate self, my daughter said to me, "Remember that time you yelled at us? Mommy, it was because of the medication. You acted weird." Out of the mouths of babes. . . . In regard to these low moments, all I can say is: Apologize, apologize, apologize. Loves means being able to say you are sorry.

Although your friends and family will likely want to support you during therapy, in all probability, they will be clueless about how to do so effectively. People may tiptoe around you, leaving you to feel lonely at the very time when you need comfort. Additionally, because HCV patients often look better than they feel, people may think you are doing better than you actually are. Being considered resilient is fine, most of the time. There will be days, however, when your insides feel like mush and those around you expect you to perform like an athlete, which can be extremely frustrating.

Good communication can make a huge difference. By keeping quiet and maintaining a tough exterior, you may think that you're making life easier for your family and friends; but if you're only pretending to feel well, sooner or later the truth will surface. Moreover, holding your feelings inside tends to lead to all sorts of emotional problems and stress-related medical issues. Nevertheless, it is very tempting to remain silent, as opening up often carries the fear of unleashing an unstoppable flood of emotions. Truthfully, though, your loved ones can sense when you are holding information from them. Feelings always find other ways to express themselves. In the end, clamming up seldom serves a purpose.

I am a person who recoils when people are overly sympathetic. During treatment, I wanted to be left alone and didn't want my family to worry about me. On really hard days, however, I wanted my family to take over the tasks I couldn't perform, and expected them to figure out what I needed and when I needed it. I learned the hard way that mind reading is not an effective form of communication. Talk to your loved ones about your illness and treatment. Give them literature on the subject. Tell them about the common side effects of therapy, including mood swings, anger, fatigue, and difficulty concentrating. Reassure them that when the treatment is over, you will go back to your old self, although not immediately. Let them know how they can support you.

Unfortunately, even with the lines of communication open, your friends and family may feel helpless. It may help to invite those closest to you to participate in your treatment process. Ask a family member or friend to accompany you to medical appointments. This has the added value of providing an extra set of ears, which is a great way to be sure you don't miss any pertinent medical information. If you attend a support group that allows visitors, ask friends and family members to attend a meeting with you. Better yet, see if your community offers a support group for caregivers of people undergoing HCV therapy. When HCV caregivers have their own group, it allows them to connect with others who understand how difficult it can be to live with HCV treatment patients. Finally, it may also reassure your loved ones to speak to someone who has completed therapy. It may be enormously relieving for them to hear another patient's experience, recognize the similarities in regard to your situation, and understand that, at some point, life will return to normal.

If your primary relationships are suffering in spite of all efforts to the contrary, consider counseling. Counseling can streamline the communication process and give all parties a chance to be heard. Most medical insurance covers the cost of family counseling, but you may need to contact your provider first for prior authorization or a referral. Most importantly, you must resist the temptation to isolate yourself. Make plans with family and friends. Go for a walk or a drive. Take in a movie or attend a local sporting event. Regularly schedule activities, and attend even if you don't really feel like showing up.

There may be days, however, when you won't be able to push yourself, and deep down, you'll know that if you are around people it won't be good for you or them. At these times, just be honest. You don't need a long, fancy explanation. Reassure your loved ones that it has nothing to do with them, and that you need to rest. Let them know that you'll speak up if you require anything.

## SEX LIFE

As discussed in the previous chapter, HCV medication may alter your body's sexual response. This side effect may or may not upset you. For instance, if you are in the mood for sex but cannot maintain an erection, you may become extremely frustrated. On the other hand, if you are in the midst of a bout of nausea, sex may be the furthest thing from your mind. Regardless of how you feel, your partner will probably not be thrilled if sexual activity drops off or stops. Additionally, if you have to use barrier contraception after years of unprotected sex, this may also be a nuisance. Reassure your partner that the problems are due to the HCV medication and have nothing to do with your feelings. Remind your loved one that the change is temporary, and that things will return to normal in the weeks and months following the end of treatment. Tell your partner that you still care, even if you may not always show it. By communicating properly, you may discover that your partner is comfortable foregoing sex for a while, as long as you maintain some emotional intimacy.

The bottom line is to be as open and honest as possible. Even if you don't want to engage in sex, be as affectionate as you can. When treatment is over, you'll want your partner there to celebrate its conclusion with you. While you will likely owe your loved one more than just a candlelit dinner, sharing a romantic meal is a good way to rekindle your sexual spark.

> *Sexuality is a private matter, but it is also a medical one. If you and your partner are having sexual problems, discuss this with you medical provider. If you need more help than your physician can offer, ask for a referral to a sex therapist or specialist.*

## CHOOSING A SUPPORT GROUP

There are few better experts on the subject of HCV medication than those who have been through treatment. Thankfully, HCV therapy patients are often eager to share survival tips that you won't get during a ten-minute medical appointment—a fact that makes attending a support group the best way to receive reliable information and encouragement.

Some groups are educationally oriented, providing literature, guest speakers, and other forms of information. Other groups may focus on the emotional side of the experience. If possible, look for a group that offers a little something for everyone. A group that is strictly educational might not meet the needs of someone who is simply scared, while a group that focuses strictly on feelings may be inappropriate for someone who wants to discuss medical facts and resources. As long as a group is built on a solid foundation of information, though, you should derive some benefit from it, so find one and give it a try.

Some support groups permit anyone to attend, including family and friends of people on HCV therapy, while others are open only to those who are undergoing treatment. There are community-based groups, as well as groups offered by a specific agency, individual, or group of medical providers. Some groups allow you to drop in at your discretion, while others encourage regular attendance. Some groups are ongoing, while others are held only for a limited number of weeks. All support groups, however, should offer confidentiality and anonymity.

To locate a group, talk to your medical provider. Some physicians offer meetings exclusively to their patients. Additionally, you may look for support through your local pharmacy, community health library, employer, or insurance company. Finally, ask your fellow HCV patients if they are aware of any meetings.

Of course, you may already belong to a supportive organization of some kind, such as a church, twelve-step program, or community group. It may be helpful to share information about your health with members of such groups. One benefit of doing so is that other people may reveal a familiarity with the subject, or even with other HCV patients, which can be extremely comforting. One possible disadvantage of exposing your condition in this setting, however, is the previously discussed stigma. People may gossip or distance themselves from you. Most times, though, people are supportive and helpful.

If you cannot find a support group in your home town, consider an online one. One benefit of Internet support groups is that there are so many of them. If you don't like one group, you can easily find another. Web-based support, however, can be a double-edged sword, with both useful and harmful aspects. For example, it is much more anonymous than in-person groups, which makes it easier for people to say things that they may not say during face-to-face discussions. This open communication can foster genuine compassion, which is a good thing, but it can also lead people to say whatever they'd like without regard for the consequences, which can result in feelings getting seriously hurt. Another problem with online conversation is that it lacks the element of body language. Communication is more than the spoken word; it involves gestures, facial expressions, and other physical cues, all of which are missing online. When you read words on a page, you hear the message in your own voice, adding meaning and interpretation from your own perspective that may not have been intended by the writer.

> *Some support groups are better than others, whether they are online or community-based. Some groups are positive and upbeat, while others are tragically negative. The quality of support groups is influenced by its leadership as well as its regular members. Try a group a few times, and if it doesn't feel supportive, look for another one.*

The immediacy of the Internet is another issue. When you discuss issues in person, the act of listening to others allows you time to think before you speak. This delay doesn't necessarily occur within online chat rooms. It is easy to type out a quick response and hit the send key without really thinking about it, which may result in regret. I urge you to practice restraint online, particularly if you are involved in an emotional conversation. Don't press the reply button for twenty-four hours. This will give you a chance to review your message before you send it. You might also ask someone you trust to read what you've written before you post it.

Whether face-to-face or online, support groups tend to attract people who are having problems, so if your aim is to pick the brains of patients who aren't experiencing side effects in the hope of learning their secret, you may be disappointed. Keep in mind, though, that many people find solutions to their problems through these groups and then stick around to help others. Before you know it, you too will be assisting others as they struggle with HCV therapy. In doing so, you are sure to discover that giving support feels even better than receiving it.

## ▢ THE BOTTOM LINE

Although HCV treatment will likely change every aspect of your life for a while, there are ways to manage it while maintaining a strong work life, social life, and romantic life. It may feel as though your body is being broken down at times, but you don't have to feel as though your entire world is being broken down, too. You may not feel the need to disclose your therapy to your employer, but there are protective measures afforded you if you do. Your family, friends, and partner may not know how to act or react towards you at first, but these barriers can be overcome with open and honest communication. And if you feel lost and in need of an experienced helping hand, support groups are out there to lend assistance both educationally and emotionally, the benefits of which can spill over into every part of your life, seeing you through to the end of therapy. If you feel overwhelmed and unsure about how to treat life's important situations, use the following sugges-tions as a reminder.

❏ Do not assume that HCV treatment will make you unable to work. See how you react to HCV medication before making job-related decisions.

❏ Working may help you endure treatment, rather than interfere with it. You may, however, need to modify your responsibilities or hours in order to perform adequately.

❏ You do not have to disclose your illness to anyone, but you may want to tell certain people about your HCV treatment in order to explain your possible mood swings and weakness.

❏ If you want protection under the Americans with Disabilities Act (ADA), you must let your employer know about your condition.

Your medical provider will need to write a letter of explanation for your personnel files.

❏ Stigma is an unfortunate component of disclosing your HCV. Never judge yourself for having the virus, no matter how you caught it.

❏ If you work in an occupation in which there is the potential for blood-to-blood contact, protect yourself and others by learning safety precautions.

❏ Try to communicate openly and honestly with family and friends.

❏ If you want to improve your communication skills, work with a counselor.

❏ Show appreciation for the support you receive.

❏ Tell your medical provider if you are having sexual problems.

❏ Let your partner know that changes in your sex life reflect the effects of HCV treatment, and not a lack of affection.

❏ A good HCV support group may make all the difference in the world, offering tips on how to ease your treatment experience.

❏ If you can't find a support group in your community, look for a web-based group.

Most importantly, remember that you don't have to go through this experience alone. Look for support in as many places as possible, and allow yourself to *be* supported.

# — 7 —

# WHAT TO DO WHEN HCV TREATMENT IS OVER

*You play the hand you're dealt.*
*I think the game's worthwhile.* —CHRISTOPHER REEVE

Patients often assume that they will immediately bounce back to being their old selves once therapy ends. When they don't, they fear that something is wrong, which is why it will help you to know what to expect when HCV treatment is over. Post-treatment recovery isn't perfectly linear; you may feel well for a while, followed by a day or more of feeling lousy. Perhaps you'll feel tired, achy, or depressed. Some people say that they feel like they are "coming down with something," but no illness ever materializes. These hard days can be discouraging and confusing, but they always pass.

Presumably, your last dose of medication will be ribavirin or a DAA, as most medical providers prescribe a week of oral medication following the last peginterferon injection. Typically, patients begin to feel better about a month after this dose, although some notice improvement in as little as two weeks. Patients continue to recover gradually, experiencing ups and downs, and returning to normal in approximately one to six months. Although the process sometimes takes longer, very few patients report a recovery time of over a year. But remember, there is more than just your physical state to consider—there is your psychological state as well. It may take more time than you think to improve your attitude, so don't worry if you aren't as excited as you thought you'd be once therapy is over.

> *Be patient with yourself when your body doesn't immediately return to normal at the end of treatment. You will need time to recover after such a taxing experience.*

Towards the end of my HCV treatment, I marked the weeks, days, and hours until the final dose, like a kid bound for Disneyland. I thought I would feel ecstatic. I thought I would experience that mixture of joy and relief normally reserved for the last day of school. By the time I reached the finish line, though, the end felt anticlimactic. Truthfully, I could hardly muster any excitement; I was too tired to feel happy or relieved. I was glad it was over, but not in a joyful sense; I was glad because I was losing stamina. Treatment was like hiking up a steeper hill than I had anticipated; I was so ready for it to be done that I didn't immediately enjoy the accomplishment of its completion. I am still surprised that it took so long to appreciate what I'd done, but I appreciated it eventually, and it felt great.

Your experience without HCV medication is just as important as your experience on the drugs. This chapter discusses what to do during the six months that follow your last dose, and what to do after you learn the final results of treatment.

## AWAITING RESULTS

As stated in Alexandre Dumas' classic novel *The Count of Monte Cristo*, all human wisdom is summed up in two words —"Wait and hope." These two words can also describe the six-month period that follows your last dose of HCV medication. If you can remain free of HCV for at least this amount of time, your doctor will deem the result a sustained virologic response. The word cure might not be used, but that is essentially what this response means. So how can you maximize your chance of remaining virus free for six months? First and foremost, abstain from alcohol and drugs. I did not drink a sip of alcohol because I wanted to make sure I followed instructions as perfectly as possible. I knew that if I drank even a teaspoon of booze and the virus came back, the guilt would haunt me for the rest of my life. Drinking alcohol seemed too big a risk. Generally, you should keep the healthful habits you adopted in preparation for and during HCV therapy. Any weight lost while undergoing treatment usually returns, so keep drinking lots of water, eating well, and exercising in order to stay trim. Most of the patients I've worked with dropped pounds during treatment only to gain them back and then some. Because I didn't want to return to the size I was before therapy, I was careful about what I ate once my appetite came back, and increased my exercise level. As my energy rose, I used that momentum to exercise even more. In addition to staying healthy, there are a few more points to consider once your therapy ends and you are awaiting the results.

## Be Careful Stopping Other Medication

If you have been taking antidepressants, thyroid pills, or any other type of medication along with your HCV drugs, do not stop using them without talking to your doctor first. The use of antidepressants should be discontinued slowly and under your doctor's supervision. Similarly, thyroid medication should not be stopped without laboratory testing and medical guidance. I have seen patients cease the use of all pharmaceuticals when their therapy came to a close, only to experience the unintended consequences of doing so, including severe depression, mental confusion, and fatigue.

## Maintain Safety Precautions Against Transmission

You may wonder if you still need to be cautious about blood-to-blood contact after therapy ends. It is best to remain vigilant. There is still the possibility of transmitting the disease to others. Maintain the same safety precautions you used throughout therapy until you are certain that the virus has been eliminated from your system. It is especially important to continue using contraception to protect against pregnancy. The strong warnings about ribavirin's potential to cause fetal abnormalities and fetal death remain in effect for six months following the last dose of HCV medication. These guidelines also apply to female partners of men who have been treated. Do not take any chance in the matter.

## Return to Regular Life Slowly

You may feel like making up for lost time by scheduling a bunch of activities as soon as treatment ends, but you shouldn't jump back into your old schedule until you see how you feel. Make gradual changes to your life; after all, you will have been through a lot by the time therapy is over. If you are on medical leave from your job, your physician may even suggest that you work only part-time for the first month of your return.

## Don't Wait to Celebrate

All too often, patients wait for the final lab results before celebrating their achievement. As important as those final results are, the real accomplishment is the completion of treatment. I think it is important to find a way to acknowledge this accomplishment once everything is said and done, whatever the results may be. You will have dedicated a large chunk of your life to therapy, and I recommend that you honor the experience in whatever alcohol-free manner brings you pleasure.

One productive way to celebrate this milestone is to dispose of all your needles and syringes. It feels good to clear away the reminders of treatment. Your medical provider or pharmacist will tell you how to safely dispose of treatment-related items, including leftover medication, if any.

*Some patients schedule a vacation after their treatment is over. This is a great way to begin the healing process.*

## Thank Your Supporters

Once your HCV therapy is over, don't forget to acknowledge the support you received from your family and friends throughout treatment. Most patients don't go through the experience alone; they are helped along by their loved ones. Some family members make great sacrifices in the process. You can show your appreciation with a simple "thank you" spoken from the heart.

*If you used a support group during treatment, continue that relationship. The waiting period after therapy ends is an emotional time. Support groups can help you deal with these feelings. Besides, you can give back to the group by sharing advice with others who have yet to undergo treatment.*

## TESTING NEGATIVE FOR HCV

If HCV is undetectable by your six-month post-treatment appointment, you will have achieved the most desired outcome: a complete and permanent response. As you know, some experts will say you are cured, while others will prefer to use the term "sustained virologic response." Whatever your physician calls it, the result means you are free of HCV, and as long as you don't engage in activities that risk a second exposure to the virus, it is almost certain that you will remain free of HCV for the rest of your life.

Of course, you may feel unsure about the permanence of testing negative for HCV. If your doctor uses words such as "sustained response," "probably," and "likely" in association with your outcome, you will understandably feel insecure. You may wonder why your medical provider won't specifically say you're cured, which would officially put your mind at ease. These are normal thoughts. Even when your liver specialist pronounces the virus undetectable and refers you back to your primary care provider, you may need more reassurance before you completely accept that HCV is truly gone. You may want more viral load testing, repeated at six-month intervals a couple more times. Your medical provider will tell you how often you will need to be retested, if at all. If you had cirrhosis or bridging fibrosis, you may need to undergo a few other exams, such as an abdominal ultrasound and blood work for elevated alpha-fetoprotein (AFP). Assuming that you do not have another form of liver disease, you should not need any more liver biopsies. If you acquired diabetes, a thyroid problem, or any other medical condition during treatment, you will need regular follow-ups.

It is important to recall that you will still have antibodies for HCV even if you test negative for the virus. The presence of HCV antibodies merely indicates that you were once exposed to the virus. If you have been denied health or life insurance because of your HCV and wish to reapply once you test negative for the virus, please note that you may be refused a second time due to the presence of these antibodies. If this happens, ask your medical provider to write a letter to your insurance company on your behalf that explains the reason for these antibodies and certifies you officially free of the disease.

It is possible to experience a bit of an identity crisis after you clear HCV from your system. Having lived as an HCV patient for so long, you might ask, "Who am I now that I don't have HCV?" In time, you will know how to answer this question. Certain people, such as Alan Franciscus, remain active in the HCV field. The founder of the Hepatitis C Support Project, Alan continues to devote his life to helping others with HCV, although he has been free of the disease since 2003.

*Now that HCV is permanently gone, you may wonder if you can drink alcohol. There are no clear recommendations on the subject, so it is best to discuss it with your medical provider. Personally, it makes sense to me to avoid anything that might hurt your liver after you've worked so hard to rid yourself of HCV.*

# TESTING POSITIVE FOR HCV

Despite having done your very best, you may test positive for HCV six months after treatment ends. The medical label for this result is "responder-relapser," but I call it an "unappreciated victory." It takes amazing determination to go through treatment, wait six months, and then hear that HCV is still there. If you learn that the virus remains in your system, you may feel anger and frustration. You will have invested a tremendous amount of time and energy in treatment. You may have dealt with side effects that were worse than you'd expected. You may also feel guilt or blame, or begin to question your every action during therapy, wishing you had eaten healthier foods, gotten more exercise, or extended your treatment. This wishing can become a bigger burden than having HCV. If you become overwhelmed by this feeling, find a way to let it go. As you may have noticed, I derive inspiration and strength from the words of others. In this case, I would quote Auguste Rodin by saying, "Nothing is a waste of time if you use your experience wisely."

Needless to say, testing positive for HCV after going through treatment is a huge disappointment. You may wonder, "Why me?" This is a question to which there is no answer, so don't ask it. Instead, practice acceptance. Try to find the blessings of having the virus. Most likely, HCV will have made you take better care of yourself. The experience of treatment may have led you to discover inner strengths and tools that enrich your life immensely. Moreover, you will be able to show understanding to other HCV patients who do not experience a cure. You won't be alone. There are already several hundred thousand HCV patients out there for whom therapy did not yield a sustained response. This does not mean that therapy didn't do them any good. Non-responders often have improved post-treatment liver biopsies, sometimes going from moderate damage to no damage. In general, a large number of patients feel significantly better after treatment than they had prior to treatment.

After sorting out your feelings, you may ask yourself, "What's next?" Basically, you should live your life as you always have with

HCV, guarding your health, abstaining from alcohol, and taking measures to make sure you don't transmit the virus to others. Your medical practitioner will recommend guidelines for continual follow-ups, including laboratory and diagnostic tests to monitor you for cirrhosis, cancer, and other possible complications of the disease. Your biggest question may be whether or not to try more treatment. Some patients need a break from even thinking about this question after their first attempt, let alone actually starting treatment right away. Others feel that there is no time like the present, and dive back into a therapy again, varying the medication regimen to fit their new medical profile.

## CONSIDERING FUTURE HCV TREATMENT

If you still have HCV after therapy, you may wonder about the availability of new drugs for future treatment. There are usually a number of drugs in various stages of development (see the inset on page 140), any of which might hold the promise of successfully defeating HCV. Your next question may be, "Should I have waited for one of these new, possibly better drugs instead of using the medication that was available to me at the time?" The answer is no. There is always a new drug around the corner, but until that drug is approved, it is a dream rather than a reality. If your chances were good with established medication, why should you have risked them by waiting to try an unknown drug?

Having said this, I recommend that you always discuss the latest developments in HCV therapy with your medical provider. The HCV drugs presently available are excellent, but there are other good ones in the pipeline. If the wait is short, and your medical provider recommends it, holding off on a second round of therapy won't likely hinder your health. If you are hoping to avoid peginterferon altogether, however, this scenario is not likely to happen anytime soon. Like telaprevir and boceprevir, most of the drugs in development are used in combination with ribavirin and peginterferon.

There are a number of HCV drugs in various stages of testing, with preliminary data showing encouraging response rates. Some of them are being tested for use with peginterferon and ribavirin, some for use only with ribavirin, and even a few for use without any other medication. So far, all look like improvements, with some treatments achieving very high success rates. The possibilities seem unlimited. Each new drug means a new form of treatment, and the chance to cure more patients. I truly believe it is just a matter of time before every HCV patient can be rid of the virus.

## Taking Part in a Clinical Trial

If you are interested in trying an HCV drug that is not yet on the market, or you cannot afford HCV medication at the moment, you may want to consider participating in a clinical trial. These research studies, however, should not be entered into casually. Thoroughly investigate any study you wish to join, making sure it has been approved by an Institutional Review Board (IRB). An IRB is a multidisciplinary group that includes medical professionals such as physicians, nurses, and pharmacists, along with non-medical community representatives. The principal goal of an IRB is to protect patients' rights. You should also receive a document called an *informed consent form*, which provides extensive details about the clinical trial. Be aware that as a volunteer, you have the right to drop out of the study at any time. Clinical trials are usually conducted at major medical centers, but they sometimes occur in smaller community settings. Because eligibility requirements can be very restrictive, you may be turned down for a study. If this should happen, try to find another study with different enrollment criteria, or wait until one opens up.

*It is normal to feel strong feelings such as anger or depression if you don't have a permanent response to treatment. But if this reaction doesn't pass or is so strong that it interferes with your ability to enjoy life, you may need professional help. Your medical provider can refer you to a behavioral health expert.*

In some studies, each volunteer receives a variation of the same medication. In other studies, a segment of the subjects receives a *placebo*, or non-medicated version of the treatment, while the remaining subjects take the actual drug for comparison. These days, though, most HCV medication trials pit the test drug against current treatment. Researchers seek to discover if the new medication is as good as or better than available drugs. In addition, they want to find out if it is safer, and if treatment with the drug would be shorter and more tolerable. If it doesn't make treatment any easier, researchers need to know if the drug produces better end results than traditional therapy, which might justify moving the product forward.

When considering a clinical trial, you should always weigh the risks against the rewards. Risks and downsides of research studies include the following possibilities.

- Appointments and record-keeping may be very time-consuming.

- Treatment may not be effective.

- You may experience adverse reactions or side effects.

- You may not receive the new drug being studied.

While these matters may sound troublesome, joining a clinical trial may still be worthwhile in light of the following potential benefits.

- Medication and medical care are generally free or less expensive.

- You may feel a sense of satisfaction from helping medical science.

- You may gain early access to the new drug being studied.

- You will have ample time with and access to a medical team that monitors you closely and provides numerous follow-ups.

If you want to try an HCV drug that is still being tested, try to find one that is in phase III or IV of clinical trials. By the time a test drug gets to these phases, a lot more is known about it, including many of its benefits and side effects. Personally, I wouldn't join a study that was in phase I or II unless I had a really solid reason to do so, such as a deep desire to help science, or advanced HCV and no better options.

If you have learned as much as you possibly can about a particular research study and still can't decide whether or not to participate in it, take a piece of paper and write down the answers to the following questions.

❑ What is the purpose of the study?

❑ What drug or drugs are being tested?

❑ Will a placebo be used? If so, what are the chances of receiving the test drug versus the placebo? If you receive the placebo, will you be offered the test drug at the end of the trial period?

❑ If the study involves a placebo, when can you expect to know if you received the placebo or the study drug?

❑ What phase of study has the drug reached? If the trial is in an early phase, how many humans have received the medication? What is known about the animal studies that used the drug?

❑ What side effects can you expect from the study drug? Are there any serious risks? What treatment would you receive if you were harmed during the study?

❑ What are the potential benefits of your participation in the study?

❑ What other options are open to you if you do not participate in the trial?

❑ Will you receive lab tests or other diagnostic tests throughout the research? If so, how often?

❑ Will you be told the results during the study, or will the results be revealed after the end of the trial?

❑ What are your responsibilities as a participant?

❑ How long does the study last? How many visits are required? Are appointments at specific times, or is the schedule flexible? Are there any other expectations that will require your time and effort?

❑ Where is the study being conducted?

❑ What should you tell your family and coworkers regarding your participation in the trial?

❑ Will you continue to see your regular physician if you participate in the study?

❑ Will you incur any costs?

❑ How many subjects will participate in the study?

❑ Will you be able to continue taking your regular medications or supplements (including prescription and over-the-counter medications, vitamins, minerals, and herbs)?

By reconsidering the facts of a study and having them written down in front of you, your thoughts on the matter should become clearer, helping you confidently settle on a decision.

## The Phases of a Clinical Trial

If a new HCV drug passes the test tube and animal research stages of development, it may be allowed to proceed to human testing, known as clinical trials. Typically, a clinical trial of a new HCV medication consists of three to four phases.

- **Phase I.** This phase establishes the safety and tolerability of the drug, as well its dosage ranges and side effects. It involves a small number—usually between twenty and eighty—of healthy subjects (people with no known disease), but it may also use participants with HCV.

- **Phase II.** Phase II investigates whether the drug is an effective treatment and collects data on risks and side effects. It uses a small number of volunteers, generally in the range of several hundred.

- **Phase III.** This stage of the trial determines the effectiveness and safety of the drug, enrolling hundreds to thousands of subjects. If all goes well in this phase, the drug is submitted for FDA approval.

- **Phase IV.** Phase IV takes place after the drug has been approved by the FDA. The scope of this phase may vary, depending on the goal of the research. For instance, a Phase IV study may look at HCV in a particular ethnic or age group. Additionally, a researcher may want to study subjects with comorbidity, which is the presence of one or more diseases along with the primary disease.

Each phase takes years to complete, and roughly five of every thousand compounds tested receive FDA approval. For a frame of reference, it took approximately four years before peginterferon was approved, and another nine years before we saw the introduction of triple therapy with DAAs. In light of these facts, when looking at drugs that are in trials, start with those in Phase III.

*Approximately eighteen people die each day while waiting for the right organ to become available for transplant. You can make a difference by becoming an organ donor.*

## BLOOD AND ORGAN DONATION

People with a history of HCV, whether the disease is active or resolved, may not donate blood to a blood bank. Occasionally, though, scientists require blood from HCV patients for research purposes. If you live near a large university—generally one with a medical school or research labs—and are interested in being a blood donor, find out if it is conducting hepatitis C research. If it is, there is a decent chance that your blood can be put to good use.

Unlike blood donation, HCV patients can donate much-needed organs and tissues. If your infection is active, your organs won't be

141

given to healthy individuals, but they may help another HCV patient. Due to the shortage of donated organs available, transplant centers offer organs harvested from HCV-positive donors to HCV patients who might otherwise die without them. In addition to transplantation purposes, medical science also requires organs—and whole bodies, in fact—for educational purposes. I still give thanks for the precious cadaver that was donated to my anatomy class. The best way to become an organ and tissue donor is to discuss your preferences with your loved ones and register with your state. Most states offer organ donor registration at the time you acquire or renew a driver's license or identification card. Some states even have web-based donor registries. (See the Resources on page 148.)

## THE BOTTOM LINE

The completion of HCV treatment should not be a signal for you to abandon the healthful habits you picked up as a result of undergoing therapy. This fact is particularly crucial during the six-month period that follows your last dose of medication, when the success or failure of therapy is uncertain. Whether or not the program eliminates the virus from your system, you should continue to take care of yourself; your body will be better off if you do. In addition to this advice, here are a few final suggestions to recall when you finish treatment:

❑ Continue to practice birth control and abstain from alcohol as you await the results of your treatment.

❑ If your HCV is undetectable six months after your last dose of medication, you are essentially cured. There is only a 0.5-percent chance that HCV will return.

❑ If you test positive for HCV six months after your last dose of medication, you will need medical follow-ups at regular intervals.

❑ If you are still HCV positive after treatment, it is perfectly normal to feel angry or depressed, or have other painful feelings. If these emotions begin to interfere with your ability to function on a day-to-day basis, however, consider seeking the help of a professional.

❏ Even people with a history of HCV may donate their organs upon death. With so many patients on transplant waiting lists, becoming an organ donor can really make a difference.

If HCV therapy doesn't work for you, it is not the end of the road. This is perhaps the most important point to remember. There are many drugs in the research pipeline that are accumulating impressive and encouraging clinical trial data. Clinical trials provide advance access to new drugs in development, and may be an option if you do not have a permanent response to HCV treatment. Stay abreast of the latest information and consider giving therapy another shot.

# CONCLUSION

*When you get in a tight place and everything*
*goes against you, until it seems as if you could*
*not hold on a minute longer, never give up then,*
*for that is just the place and time when*
*the tide will turn.* —HARRIET BEECHER STOWE

H CV is a curable condition. Thanks to the latest treatments, four out of five HCV patients can spend the rest of their lives free of the disease. I wrote this book because I believe that just about everyone can get through HCV treatment with the right guidance. Aside from having personally undergone treatment, I have helped many patients through therapy. This guide is the result of not only my experience, but also the experiences of numerous others. I am counting on the information in this book to work for both you and me. Yes, for me too. You see, I still have hepatitis C. When I went through treatment in 2003, the odds of being permanently cured were only about 50 percent. Unfortunately, my result fell within the 50 percent of unsuccessful outcomes.

Initially, treatment made me quite anemic. In response to this side effect, my medical provider slightly reduced my ribavirin dosage. What was not known at the time was that a reduction in ribavirin during the first twelve weeks of therapy decreases the chance of permanently eliminating the virus. A better choice would have been to prescribe epoetin alfa (Epogen, Procrit) to stimulate red blood cell production. While epoetin alpha has some serious side effects and may not be for every HCV patient, I was a good candidate, which was proven by the fact that my doctor eventually recommended the medication. The adjustment, however, likely came too late. Hindsight is, of course, 20/20.

Those who saw me through treatment, including my patients, felt terrible for me. Except for me, everyone I knew who had completed at least forty-eight weeks of treatment was successfully cured. But I don't feel bad about what happened. My liver biopsy went from stage two (moderate damage) to stage zero (no damage), and once the side effects of the medication wore off, I felt significantly better than I had prior to therapy. Most of all, I was proud that I had tried.

At this point, I would like to apologize for hiding the outcome of my treatment. The decision to withhold the information until the end of the book was not undertaken lightly. I treasure the trust of my patients, and I hope to gain the trust of my readers. But had you focused on my outcome rather than the facts of HCV therapy, you might have missed the opportunity of a lifetime: a chance to live without hepatitis C.

Remember that you are not alone in this journey. Many others will be joining you, myself included. Yes, I am going to do treatment again. In light of the availability of better drugs, the use of response-guided therapy, and the possibility of only twenty-four weeks of treatment, I can't let the opportunity slip by. Besides, the chance of successful therapy decreases with age, and I am not getting any younger.

As I write these words, I am preparing for HCV treatment. I am following the same guidelines that you will follow, all of which can be found in this book. I am concentrating on optimizing my health so that I may start on a firm foundation. My doctor and I are discussing which drug regimen is best for me and determining my start date. When that date arrives, I will go through the necessary lab tests and medical appointments. I will get in touch with my insurance company and pharmacy, and sign up for the free support offered by the drug manufacturers. I will attend my community's HCV support group. After I receive my medication, I will review the instructions, making sure I haven't overlooked anything.

Once I start treatment, I will develop a system to remind myself when to take my medication. I will use the techniques and methods at my disposal to manage side effects and live my life. If I neglect my health and mental well-being, I will count on my support system to get me back on track. When treatment is over, I will await the results. Because the outcome is not as important as the effort, I will claim my victory the day I take my last dose of medication, long before I know the result of treatment. This virus will not determine my success; I will measure my success by what I put into treatment, not what I got out of it. You can claim the same victory, and you will. While you imagine the sense of freedom that comes with eliminating HCV from your body, know that real freedom occurs the moment you choose to step into the battle against the virus. The odds are in your favor, so carry the best weapons of all: patience and determination. Hang on to them, and no matter what, don't ever give up.

# RESOURCES

While a diagnosis of hepatitis C may be frightening and confusing, there are numerous federal organizations, private foundations and support groups, informational websites, and knowledgeable advocates that can help you gain confidence and clarity in the face of this adversity. Listed below are some of the best resources available to HCV patients.

## ALCOHOL, TOBACCO, AND SUBSTANCE ABUSE

**Alcoholic Anonymous (AA)**
(212) 870-3400
www.alcoholics-anonymous.org
*In addition to providing information on AA's twelve-step program, this website addresses a number of alcohol-related issues and lists meeting locations.*

**Centers for Disease Control and Prevention**
(800) CDC-INFO (800-232-4636)
www.cdc.gov/tobacco
*This section of the CDC's website is a good resource for people who wish to stop using tobacco products.*

**Narcotic Anonymous (NA)**
(818) 773-9999
www.na.org
*This organization provides assistance to narcotics addicts, helping them quit drugs and stay in recovery.*

**National Institute on Drug Abuse**
www.nida.nih.gov
*This government website presents scientific facts about alcohol, drugs, and tobacco.*

**Substance Abuse and Mental Health Services Administration**
(877) SAMHSA-7 (877-726-4727)
www.samhsa.gov
*This website is designed to help people afflicted with mental illness and substance abuse problems.*

# CLINICAL TRIALS

## CenterWatch
www.centerwatch.com
*This resource helps patients find clinical trials and outlines information on drugs and drug research.*

## ClinicalTrials
www.clinicaltrials.gov
*This website is a database of federally and privately run clinical trials. It explains the goal of each listed trial, who may join the study, and where it is located.*

## Clinical Trial Connection
www.clinicalconnection.com
*This website is another informative resource for patients looking for clinical trials.*

## HCV Advocate
www.hcvadvocate.org
*Find the latest updates on drugs in clinical testing by clicking on the* hcv DRUG pipeline *link, or learn more about HCV research by clicking on the* hcsp Fact Sheets *link and reading* Hepatitis C: Making Sense of Hepatitis C Research and Medical Literature.

## National Institutes of Health
(301) 496-4000
www.nih.gov
*This government agency provides information on a wealth of health topics.*

# COMPLEMENTARY AND ALTERNATIVE MEDICINE

## ConsumerLab
www.consumerlab.com
*This organization tests the quality of dietary supplements and maintains a database of results. While some of the website's information is free, there is a membership fee for total access.*

## Doc Misha's Chicken Soup Chinese Medicine
www.docmisha.com
*This website is packed with information on Chinese medicine, including acupuncture, herbs, and nutrition, and how it may be used by HCV patients.*

## Drug and Supplement Interactions Checker
www.drugs.com/drug_interactions.php
*This online tool enables you to see if your drugs and supplements are compatible with each other.*

## HCV Advocate
www.hcvadvocate.org
*To find research on herbs and their effects on the liver, click on the* Herbal Glossary *link of this website. For more information on the subject, go to the* Fact Sheets *section and read the links listed under* Hepatitis C and Complementary and Alternative Medicine.

## Memorial Sloan-Kettering Cancer Center
www.mskcc.org/aboutherbs
*This website has an extensive database on herbs and other supplements.*

## National Center for Complementary and Alternative Medicine:

(888) 644-6226
www.nccam.nih.gov
*This website offers research-based information on complementary and alternative medicine. Be sure to order or download the* Herbs at a Glance *booklet.*

**Natural Medicines Comprehensive Database**
www.naturaldatabase.com
*This website charges its users a monthly or annual subscription, but it is worth it. The database includes evidence-based information about supplements, drugs, drug interactions, and diseases. For an additional fee, users can access ratings of commercial products.*

**New York Online Access to Health**
www.noah-health.org/en/alternative/index.html
*This website details a number of alternative healing approaches and provides links to other resources that may help you find a practitioner of complementary and alternative medicine.*

## DIAGNOSTIC TESTS

**Lab Tests Online**
www.labtestsonline.org
*This is an online resource designed to guide users through various aspects of laboratory testing.*

**MedlinePlus**
www.nlm.nih.gov/medlineplus/laboratorytests.html
*This website provides links to the latest news, research, and information concerning lab testing.*

## DISABILITY, DISCLOSURE, AND WORKPLACE ISSUES

**HCV Advocate**
www.hcvadvocate.org
*To learn about insurance and disability benefits, click on the* Benefits Column *link of this website.*

**US Benefits Information**
www.benefits.gov
*This website is the official US government resource on benefits, grants, and other assistance.*

**US Department of Justice Americans with Disability Act**
(800) 514-0301
www.ada.gov
*This government website provides links to publications and other information concerning disability issues.*

**US Department of Labor Family and Medical Leave Act**
(866) 4-USA-DOL (866-487-2365)
www.dol.gov/whd/fmla/index.htm
*This website covers the various aspects of the* Family and Medical Leave Act.

**US Department of Labor's Job Accommodation Network**
(800) 232-9675
www.askjan.org
*This website is a good source of information for patients who have questions about workplace accommodations for people with disabilities.*

**US Disability Information**
www.disability.gov
*This website is an excellent*

resource on the subject of disabilities.

US Equal Employment Opportunity Commission
(800) 669-4000
www.eeoc.gov
*This organization provides protection against discrimination in the workplace.*

# FINANCIAL ISSUES AND MEDICAL INSURANCE

Mcdicare
(800) MEDICARE (800-633-4227)
www.medicare.gov
*This website is the official US government resource on Medicare.*

Needy Meds
www.needymeds.com
*This organization is devoted to helping reduce the cost of medication.*

Partnership for Prescription Assistance
(888) 4PPA-NOW (888-477-2669)
www.pparx.org
*This program helps qualifying individuals without prescription drug coverage find free or low-cost medicine.*

Patients Access Network Foundation
(866) 316-PANF (866-316-7263)
www.panfoundation.org
*This foundation provides assistance to underinsured patients by lowering the out-of-pocket costs of prescription drugs.*

# HEALTHY LIFESTYLE AND GENERAL HEALTH

Aetna Intelihealth
www.intelihealth.com
*Provided courtesy of Aetna in association with Harvard Medical School, this website offers ways to maintain general health.*

Centers for Disease Control and Prevention
www.cdc.gov
*This website supplies a wide range of information on virtually every health-related subject.*

Cochrane Collaboration
www.cochrane.org
*This international website provides the latest evidence in healthcare research.*

Food and Drug Administration (FDA)
(888) INFO-FDA (888-463-6332)
www.fda.gov
*In addition to consumer information, this website presents the latest health-related research and information.*

HealthFinder
www.healthfinder.gov
*This website is filled with health information. It contains over fifty online check-up tools, including one that will help you create a heart-healthy diet.*

MedlinePlus
www.nlm.nih.gov/medlineplus
*Consult this resource for reliable, up-to-date health information from the National Institutes of*

*Health and the National Library of Medicine.*

## Merck Engage
www.merckengage.com
*Although a pharmaceutical company sponsors this site, the information is good and free of advertisements.*

## National Institutes of Health
www.nih.gov
*This organization offers information about many health-related topics, including liver disease.*

## PubMed
www.ncbi.nlm.nih.gov/pubmed
*Produced by the National Institutes of Health and the National Library of Medicine, this online tool contains millions of citations for biomedical literature. The PubMed Tutorials teach readers how to use this resource effectively.*

## US Department of Health and Human Services
www.hhs.gov
*This government agency's website is a gateway to multiple sources of health information.*

# HEPATITIS C

## American Association for the Study of Liver Diseases
www.aasld.org
*This group is the largest professional organization devoted to liver diseases in the US. Its HCV Practice Guidelines are worth reading.*

## American Liver Foundation

www.liverfoundation.org
*This organization is devoted to raising awareness of liver diseases and publishes an online quarterly magazine,* Liver Health Today.

## Caring Ambassadors Hepatitis C Program
www.hepcchallenge.org
*The mission of this organization is to help improve the lives of those affected by HCV.*

## HCV Advocate
www.hcvadvocate.org
*This organization promotes awareness of issues related to HCV. It provides educational information in connection with nearly every facet of HCV, along with links to many other helpful websites.*

## Hepatitis C Association
www.hepcassoc.org
*This association provides information and support to those affected by HCV.*

## Hepatitis Education Project
www.hepeducation.org
*This education-based program offers a wide range of information for those affected by HCV.*

## Hepatitis Foundation International
www.hepfi.org
*This foundation is committed to advocacy and education in connection with issues pertaining to viral hepatitis.*

## HIV and Hepatitis
www.hivandhepatitis.com
*This website provides excellent*

information on HCV as well as HIV/HCV coinfection.

## National AIDS Treatment Advocacy Project

www.natap.org
*This project offers up-to-date evidence-based news and research on HCV as well as HIV/HCV coinfection.*

## National Viral Hepatitis Roundtable

www.nvhr.org
*This group is a national coalition that comprises private, public, and volunteer organizations, all of which are acting to lessen the impact of viral hepatitis in the United States.*

## US Department of Veterans Affairs Hepatitis C Information

www.hepatitis.va.gov
*Not just for veterans, this website supplies a wide range of information on HCV for patients and providers.*

## World Hepatitis Alliance

www.worldhepatitisalliance.org
*This international non-profit organization's ultimate goal is to work with governments around the world in an effort to achieve a world without hepatitis B or C.*

## HUMOR

### Helpguide

www.helpguide.org/life/humor_laughter_health.htm
*This link discusses the health benefits of laughter and suggests ways to incorporate humor into a healthy lifestyle.*

## The Hepatitis Comics: Levity for the Liver

www.hepatitiscomics.blogspot.com
*This web address will take you to my blog, billed as "bile humor and heptainment to tickle the liver."*

## Laughter Heals Foundation

www.laughterheals.org
*This website offers jokes, stories, and articles devoted to using laughter to hasten the healing process.*

## MENTAL HEALTH

### HCV Advocate

www.hcvadvocate.org
*For multiple articles on mental health and HCV, browse the* Fact Sheets *section of this website.*

### Helpguide

www.helpguide.org
*This website addresses multiple health issues, with a special emphasis on mental health.*

### International Foundation for Research and Education for Depression

(800) 442-HOPE (800-442-4673)
www.ifred.org
*This organization offers access to self-assessment tools such as a depression test, as well as tips to manage depression.*

### Mayo Clinic

www.mayoclinic.com/health/ssris/MH00066
*While you should definitely browse the rest of this website for more mental health information, the address above will take*

you to an excellent article on depression medication.

**Medline**
www.nlm.nih.gov/medlineplus
*Click on the* Health Topics *link on this website and find general information on depression by locating the subject alphabetically on the list.*

**Mental Health America**
www.mentalhealthamerica.net
*This website provides links to multiple mental health resources.*

**National Alliance for the Mentally Ill**
800-950-NAMI (800-950-6264)
www.nami.org
*This organization is highly regarded for its mental health advocacy and educational material on the subject.*

**National Institute of Mental Health**
(866) 615-6464
www.nimh.nih.gov
*This evidence-based website is loaded with useful educational material, links, and other information related to mental health.*

# NUTRITION AND WEIGHT MANAGEMENT

**Harvard School of Public Health**
www.hsph.harvard.edu/nutrition-source/index.html
*This website is a first-rate resource on the subject of nutrition.*

**Nutrition.gov**
www.nutrition.gov
*This federal government website*

offers reliable information on food and nutrition, as well as links to interactive tools to help you make healthful choices.

**Oldways**
www.oldwayspt.org
*This organization highlights the pleasure of eating while it also educates the reader on nutrition. It offers alternative nutrition pyramids for a variety of diets, including Mediterranean, Latin, Asian, and vegetarian.*

# ORGAN DONATION

**Donate Life America**
www.donatelife.net
*This organization provides information on organ and tissue donation, including how to register as an organ donor in your state.*

# PATIENT ADVOCACY

**Hepatitis Prison Coalition**
www.hcvinprison.org
*This organization raises awareness of and provides support to prisoners with HCV or other chronic viruses.*

**Patient Advocate Foundation**
www.patientadvocate.org
*This foundation offers assistance to patients who have health-related insurance problems, medical debt, employment issues, or financial troubles.*

# PHARMACEUTICAL RESOURCES

**Genentech Access Solutions**

www.genentechaccesssolutions.com
*This website offers HCV patients
and caregivers support, information, and assistance.*

**Incivek**
(888) 552-2494 or (855) 837-8394
www.incivek.com
*Created by the drug manufacturer
Vertex, this website assists
patients who take its* Incivek
*brand of telaprevir.*

**Kadmon Pharmaceuticals**
(888) 668-3393
www.kadmon.com
*This company manufactures rib-
avirin under the name* Ribas-
phere, *and their website provides
information, resources, and assistance to HCV patients.*

**Merck CARES**
www.merck-cares.com
(866) 939-HEPC (4372)
*As the manufacturers of a number
of HCV drugs, including peginterferon* (PegIntron), *ribavirin* (Rebetol), *and boceprevir* (Victrelis),
*Merck's website ocuses on HCV
education and support. The* Merck
Patient Assistance Program *provides free medicine for eligible
patients, while the* Merck ACT
Program *helps patients find coverage for medication and reveals
ways to reduce out-of-pocket costs.*

**Pegasys and Copegus**
(877) PEGASYS (877-734-2797)
www.pegasys.com
*Created by drug manufacturer
Genentech, this website assists
patients who take its* Pegasys

*brand of peginterferon and its*
Copegus *brand of ribavirin.*

**Victrelis**
www.victrelis.com
*Created by drug manufacturer
Merck, this website assists
patients who take its* Victrelis
*brand of boceprevir.*

## PHYSICAL FITNESS

**President's Council on Fitness,
Sports and Nutrition**
www.fitncss.gov
*This government organization's web-
site presents information and links
to educational resources on fitness.*

**Shape Up America**
www.shapeup.org
*This non-profit organization's
website guides users through various aspects of fitness, including
exercise and weight control.*

**Squeeze It In**
www.squeezeitin.com
*Although this fitness program
focuses more on women, its best
feature is that it offers simple exercises that anyone can do throughout the day, anywhere, anytime.*

**United States Department of
Health and Human Services**
www.smallstep.gov
*Provided by the US government,
this resource presents tips and
facts to help people get fit, eat
better, and improve their health
in small increments.*

## PREGNANCY AND CONTRACEPTION

**Planned Parenthood**
(800) 230-PLAN (800-230-7526)
www.plannedparenthood.org
*This group is the leading sexual and reproductive healthcare advocate in the country. Among other helpful facts, this website offers information on birth control.*

**Ribavirin Pregnancy Registry**
(800) 593-2214
www.ribavirinpregnancyregistry.com
*This registry is a voluntary program that collects data on pregnancies that may have been exposed to the HCV drug ribavirin, which can occur when a female patient conceives while she or her partner is undergoing HCV treatment.*

## SIDE EFFECT MANAGEMENT

**HCV Advocate**
www.hcvadvocate.org
*For helpful advice on side effect management, go to the* Fact Sheets *section of this website and read* A Guide to Hepatitis C: Treatment Side Effect Management.

**The Combo Survival Guide from A to Z**
www.hepcsurvivalguide.org/comboguide.htm
*This resource features medically-reviewed, patient-written side effect information, presented with a bit of humor.*

## SLEEP

**American Academy of Sleep Medicine**
www.yoursleep.aasmnet.org
*This website provides dependable educational material on the subject of sleep and sleep disorders.*

**American Sleep Association**
www.sleepassociation.org
*This association is dedicated to raising awareness of sleep disorders and sleep health.*

**The National Sleep Foundation**
www.sleepfoundation.org
*This foundation's comprehensive website addresses the importance of getting adequate sleep and learning good sleep habits.*

## STRESS, MEDITATION, AND ANGER MANAGEMENT

**The American Institute of Stress**
www.stress.org
*This non-profit organization's website acts as a clearinghouse for information related to stress and its effects on health.*

**American Psychological Association**
www.apa.org
*For information on anger management, click on* Anger *under* Psychology Topics *on the opening page of this website.*

**Anger Management Techniques**
www.anger-management-techniques.org
*This website suggests anger man-*

agement methods based on Buddhist tradition.

## Free Meditation Technique
www.freemeditations.com
*This website is a gateway to many types of meditation techniques.*

## Hep C Meditations
www.hepCmeditations.org
*This website sells an instructional CD designed to help HCV patients deal with the challenges of the illness through meditation. It also offers a free download of the audio lesson 7* Minutes to Liver Health.

## The Institute of Lifestyle Medicine
www.instituteoflifestylemedicine.org
*Click on* Tools and Resources *to access useful information that can help you reduce stress and improve your health.*

## Mayo Clinic
www.mayoclinic.com
*In addition to an abundance of other health information, this website has a search engine that can help you find advice on how to deal with stress and anger.*

## Medline
www.nlm.nih.gov/medlineplus/stress.html
*This website is a good starting point to learn about stress in general and offers links to other resources on the subject.*

## Stressbusting
www.stressbusting.co.uk
*This website covers many aspects*

of stress and offers ways to eliminate stress from your life.

## World Wide Online Meditation Center
www.meditationcenter.com
*This online resource provides the basic information required to learn how to meditate.*

# SUPPORT GROUPS

## Google Groups
http://groups.google.com
*This resource can help you find online support groups; simply type "hepatitis C" in the search field.*

## HCV Advocate
www.hcvadvocate.org
*Click on the* Support Groups *link of this website to find an HCV support group meeting in your area. Additionally, click on* Fact Sheets *and read the* Hepatitis C Support Group Manual.

## Healthy Hepper
www.healthyhepper.com/events.htm
*This website lists HCV-related events and support groups.*

## Hepatitis Central
www.hepatitis-central.com/hcv/support/main.html
*Despite the excessive number of advertisements on this website, it is a good resource, offering a map designed to help HCV patients locate support groups in their area.*

## Yahoo Groups
http://groups.yahoo.com
*This resource can help you find online support groups; simply type "hepatitis C" in the search field.*

**FutureMe.org**
www.futureme.org
*This website allows you to send
encouraging emails to yourself
that will arrive in the future on a
chosen date. It is especially useful if you write your supportive
emails at the beginning of treatment, when you are at your best,
and schedule them to arrive later
in therapy, when you need the
most encouragement.*

**TRANSMISSION/PREVENTION**

**Centers for Disease Control and
Prevention**
www.cdc.gov
*In addition to the facts on hepati-
tis C prevention, this government
website offers a huge amount of
information on general health.*

**Harm Reduction Coalition**
www.harmreduction.org
*This organization advocates a set
of strategies to reduce the negative consequences of drug use,
which include both safer drug
use and abstinence.*

# GLOSSARY

**abdominal ultrasound.** A non-invasive scan that uses sound waves to produce an image of the liver and other organs in the abdomen.

**absolute neutrophil count (ANC).** Part of the Complete Blood Count, the ANC is a measurement of neutrophils, which are a type of white blood cell.

**acute hepatitis C.** The initial stage of hepatitis C, referring to the first six months of infection.

**adverse event.** An undesired effect of or reaction to treatment.

**alanine aminotransferase (ALT).** An enzyme manufactured by the liver and measured with a blood test. An elevated ALT level indicates damaged liver cells. ALT used to be known as SGPT.

**alpha-fetoprotein (AFP).** A protein found in the blood that is used to screen for certain types of cancer, including liver cancer. Hepatitis patients, however, often display elevated AFP levels without the presence of cancer.

**anemia.** Low red blood cell count, which may be caused by a number of factors.

**antibodies.** Proteins produced by the immune system after a foreign substance enters the body. Positive HCV antibodies indicate past exposure or current infection, and require further testing to determine if HCV is active. Negative HCV antibodies mean that there is no HCV infection, unless the exposure was recent. A negative result should be tested again 6 months after suspected HCV exposure.

**autoimmune disease.** A class of diseases that occur when the body's immune system mistakes part of itself as a foreign substance, causing it to attack itself.

**blind study.** A study in which subjects do not know if they are receiving the test drug or the placebo.

**boceprevir.** A protease inhibitor used to treat HCV.

**brain fog.** A term that refers to mild mental or cognitive impairment, which sometimes accompanies HCV. Brain fog is not to be confused with hepatic encephalopathy, which is much more severe.

**bridging fibrosis.** Extensive fibrosis that forms a bridge between the liver's portal tracts.

**chemistry panel.** A lab test that measures liver enzymes, electrolytes, and other chemicals in the body. Also known as a Comprehensive Metabolic Panel, it is used to assess kidney and liver function, as well as overall health.

**chronic hepatitis C.** The persistence of the hepatitis C virus, referring to an infection that lasts longer than six months.

**cirrhosis.** Severe scarring of the liver, which may be irreversible.

**clinical trials.** Research studies that analyze the safety and effectiveness of new treatments.

**combination therapy.** Therapy that uses two or more drugs in combination to improve the effectiveness of treatment. When applied to HCV, this term most often refers to the use of peginterferon plus ribavirin (PegIFN/RBV).

**comorbidity.** The presence of more than one disease, such as diabetes and HCV.

**compensated cirrhosis.** A cirrhotic liver that still functions fairly well.

**complementary and alternative medicine (CAM).** Healing practices that are used with or instead of conventional Western Medicine, such as acupuncture or chiropractics. Other terms for CAM include holistic, mind-body, and integrative medicine.

**complete blood count (CBC).** A basic lab test that measures components of the blood, including red blood cells, white blood cells, and platelets. The CBC further measures subsets of these cells including hemoglobin and neutrophils.

**contraindication.** A condition or factor that makes the use of a particular drug or treatment inadvisable.

**control group.** The group of subjects in a clinical trial who receive the current standard treatment or no active treatment, and not the new drug being studied.

**decompensated cirrhosis.** Cirrhosis that is so advanced that the liver can't perform essential functions.

**direct-acting antivirals (DAAs).** Drugs that target a specific virus, such as HCV. Also known as STAT-C or Specifically Targeted Antiviral Therapy drugs.

**double-blind, randomized, placebo-controlled study.** The highest standard of research, this study randomly assigns subjects to a group receiving the test drug or a placebo (an inactive substance). No one, not even the research team, knows who is taking the drug or the placebo.

**early virologic response (EVR).** An early response means that there is no detectable HCV after the first twelve weeks of treatment. EVR is called a negative predictor of response because it suggests who will not be cured of HCV, as 97 to 100 percent of those without an EVR will also fail to achieve a sustained response. Although an EVR is a good sign, it is not as strong as a Rapid Virologic Response (RVR).

**edema.** Swelling caused by excess fluid accumulation trapped inside body tissue.

**extrahepatic manifestations.** Symptoms of HCV that affect organs other than the liver.

**fibrosis.** Minimal to moderate damage to liver tissue. Fibrosis is not as severe as cirrhosis, and is reversible.

**Food and Drug Administration (FDA).** Responsible for the safety of food and drugs, this US government agency may approve or deny the availability of a drug to the public.

**gastroenterologist.** A physician who specializes in diseases of the digestive system, which includes the liver.

**genotype (GT).** Genetic variation in a virus. HCV has six major genotypes, labeled 1 through 6, which can have many subtypes.

**hcv viral load (HCV RNA).** A measurement of the presence and amount of the HCV virus in the blood.

**hemoglobin (Hgb).** Part of the red blood cell that carries oxygen to other parts of the body. Low hemoglobin usually indicates anemia.

**hemolytic anemia.** A type of anemia caused by the bursting of red blood cells, which is a possible side effect of ribavirin.

**hepatic encephalopathy.** Severe mental confusion that accompanies cirrhosis of the liver.

**hepatic panel.** A lab test that measures liver enzymes, or chemicals in the liver, the hepatic panel is sometimes part of a bigger battery of tests called a comprehensive metabolic panel or chemistry panel.

**hepatitis.** Inflammation of the liver that may be caused by a variety of factors, such as a virus, alcohol use, toxins, mold, obesity, or autoimmune disease.

**hepatitis A (HAV).** A viral disease that is spread primarily through oral contact with contaminated fecal matter. Although HAV and HCV are two completely different viruses, their symptoms are sometimes similar. HAV is highly infectious in its initial stages, but usually resolves itself without treatment, leaving the infected immune to it. There is an HAV vaccine.

**hepatitis B (HBV).** A viral disease spread primarily through contact with blood and other bodily fluids, HBV is sexually transmitted. HBV and HCV are completely different viruses. HBV is highly infectious in its initial stages, but usually resolves itself without treatment, leaving the infected immune to it. In some cases, however, HBV can become chronic. There is an HBV vaccine.

**hepatitis C (HCV).** A viral disease that primarily affects the liver, HCV is spread through blood-to-blood contact. There is no HCV vaccine.

**hepatocellular carcinoma.** Cancer of the liver.

**hepatologist.** A gastroenterologist who specializes in diseases of the liver.

**institutional review board (IRB).** A group that reviews and approves all research involving animal or human subjects. The IRB monitors research to ensure that the rights and welfare of research subjects are protected.

162

**interferon alfa.** A naturally occurring protein produced by the body's immune system to interfere with viral reproduction. Interferon alfa has been genetically engineered to treat HCV, modified into a version known as pegylated interferon or peginterferon.

**lichen planus.** A skin disorder that causes rash and itching. Those with HCV have a higher risk for this condition.

**liver biopsy.** A procedure that extracts tissue from the liver, usually with a hollow-core needle. The procedure is performed in an outpatient setting, using a local anesthetic and, usually, mild sedation.

**log drop.** A term used to evaluate a patient's response to treatment. The simplest way to determine a log drop is to remove the last digit of the viral load result, dropping one digit for a one-log drop, two digits for a two-log drop, and so on. So, if the viral load is 1,800,000 IU/ml, a one-log drop would be 180,000 IU/ml, and a two-log drop would be 18,000 IU/ml. A patient's goals are typically defined as certain number of log drops within a certain number of weeks of treatment.

**medical provider.** Also known as a healthcare provider, this term refers to physicians, nurse practitioners, and physician assistants (PAs).

**neutrophil.** A type of white blood cell that frequently drops to abnormal levels during HCV treatment.

**non-responder.** A label used to describe a patient whose HCV viral load remains detectable during treatment.

**pegylated interferon, or peginterferon (PegIFN).** One of the medications used to treat HCV. Peginterferon is a form of interferon alfa that has been modified in order to stay in the body longer. It requires fewer injections than unmodified interferon alfa.

**placebo.** An inactive substance used to determine the effectiveness of a test drug through comparison in a clinical trial.

**platelets.** Components of the blood that help it clot. Low platelets may be a sign of cirrhosis, but are also a common side effect of HCV treatment.

**portal tracts.** The part of the liver's structure that contains blood vessels and ducts.

**protease inhibitor.** A type of drug that interferes with the lifecycle of a virus, HCV protease inhibitors are specifically designed to stop

HCV replication by blocking the protease enzyme required for the virus to survive.

**randomization.** The process of randomly assigning clinical trial volunteers to either the control group, which receives a placebo, or the group that receives the test drug.

**rapid virologic response (RVR).** The term used to describe patients whose virus becomes undetectable early in treatment (usually the first four weeks). Patients who have an RVR are very likely to attain a sustained response, or cure.

**red blood cells (RBC).** Cells in the blood that carry oxygen to every part of the body.

**responder-relapser.** The term used in reference to HCV patients who are HCV-negative during treatment but become HCV-positive again once treatment ends.

**response-guided therapy.** This form of therapy bases its regimen on the patient's response to HCV medication and allows for adjustments to be made according to future test results.

**ribavirin (RBV).** An antiviral drug used with interferon to treat HCV infection.

**sustained virologic response (SVR).** The term used by medical providers to describe when a patient remains free of HCV for six months after treatment has stopped.

**telaprevir.** A protease inhibitor, telaprevir is one of the newest HCV treatment drugs.

**thyroid disease.** A disease affecting a small gland in the throat, which causes it to produce too much or too little thyroid hormone. HCV treatment may cause thyroid abnormities.

**triple therapy.** The use of three drugs to treat a condition. In connection with HCV, triple therapy likely refers to peginterferon, ribavirin, and a protease inhibitor.

**viral replication.** The ability of a virus to reproduce.

**virus.** A microscopic infectious particle that invades a living organism and generates copies of itself.

**white blood cell (WBC).** A type of blood cell with many components, which plays a major role in the body's immune system.

# REFERENCES

## CHAPTER 1

1. Davis, G.L, Alter M.J, El-Serag, H, et al. "Aging of hepatitis C virus (HCV)-infected persons in the United States: a multiple cohort model of HCV prevalence and disease progression." *Gastroenterology* (2010); 138: 513–521.
2. ibid.
3. ibid.
4. National Institutes of Health Consensus Development Conference Panel Statement: Management of Hepatitis C. *Hepatology* (Sept. 1997): 26(3, Suppl. 1):2S–10S.
5. Rebetol, Intron, and Rebetron product information.
6. Compilation of data from product information of peginterferon alfa-2a with ribavirin (Pegasys/Copegus) and peginterferon alfa-2b with ribavirin (PegIntron/Rebetron).
7. ibid.
8. Telaprevir (Incivek) prescribing information.
9. Telaprevir (Incivek) prescribing information.

## CHAPTER 2

1. Swain, M, Lai, M-Y, Shiffman, M.L, et al. "Durable sustained virological response after treatment with peginterferon alfa-2a (Pegasys) alone or in combination with ribavirin (Copegus): 5-year follow-up and the criteria of a cure." Program and abstracts of the

42nd Annual Meeting of the European Association for the Study of the Liver; April 11–15, 2007. Barcelona, Spain. Abstract 1.

2. Maylin, S, Martinot-Peignoux, M, Ripault, M, et al. "Sustained Virological Response Is Associated with Clearance of Hepatitis C Virus RNA and a Decrease in Hepatitis C Virus Antibody." *Liver International* (April 2009); 29(4): 511–517.

3. *Science Daily* (May 22, 2007).

4. Telaprevir (Incivek) prescribing information.

5. Package insert of peginterferon alfa-2a (Pegasys) used with ribavirin.

6. Fried, M, Shiffman, M, Reddy, R, et al. "Peginterferon alfa-2a plus Ribavirin for Chronic Hepatitis C Virus Infection." *New England Journal of Medicine* (2002); 347: 975–982.

7. Davis, G. "Monitoring of Viral Levels during Therapy of Hepatitis C." *Hepatology* (Nov. 2002); 36(5, Suppl. 1): S145–S151.

# RECOMMENDED READING

*The Anxiety and Phobia Workbook* by Edmund J. Bourne, PhD. Oakland, CA: New Harbinger Publications, Inc, 2000.

*Dr. Melissa Palmer's Guide to Hepatitis and Liver Disease* by Melissa Palmer. New York: Avery, Penguin Group Inc, 2000.

*The Gift of Fire* by Dan Caro with Steve Erwin. Carlsbad, CA: Hay House, Inc, 2010.

*Healing Hepatitis C* by Christopher Kennedy Lawford and Diana Sylvestre, MD. New York: Harper Collins, 2009.

*The Hepatitis C Help Book, Revised Edition: A Groundbreaking Treatment Program Combining Western and Eastern Medicine for Maximum Wellness and Healing* by Misha Ruth Cohen, OMD, Lac; and Robert Gish, MD; with Kalia Doner. New York: St. Martin's Griffin, 2007.

*Living with Hepatitis C, Fifth Edition: A Survivor's Guide* by Gregory T. Everson, MD, FACP. New York: Hatherleigh Press, 2009.

*Living with Hepatitis C for Dummies* by Nina L. Paul. Hoboken, NJ: Wiley Publishing, Inc, 2005.

*The Miracle of Mindfulness* by Thich Nhat Hanh. Boston: Beacon Press, 1999.

*The Promise of Sleep* by William C. Dement, MD, PhD; and Christopher Vaughan. New York: Dell Publishing, 2000.

*Teach Yourself to Meditate in 10 Simple Lessons* by Eric Harrison. Berkeley, CA: Ulysses Press, 2001.

# About the Author

Lucinda K. Porter is both a hepatitis C nurse and patient. Based on her work at Stanford University Medical Center, and as a public speaker and writer, she is recognized as an expert in the field of HCV. In addition to the many HCV guides and pamphlets she has written, Lucinda has been contributing two monthly columns to the online resource *HCV Advocate* since 1998. She lives in Grass Valley, California.

# INDEX

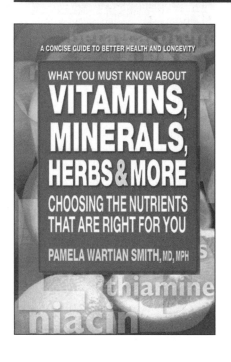

# WHAT YOU MUST KNOW ABOUT VITAMINS, MINERALS, HERBS & MORE

Choosing the Nutrients
That Are Right for You

Pamela Wartian Smith, MD, MPH

Almost 75 percent of your health and life expectancy is based on lifestyle, environment, and nutrition. Yet even if you follow a sound diet, you are probably not getting all the nutrients you need to prevent disease. In *What You Must Know About Vitamins, Minerals, Herbs & More*, Dr. Pamela Smith explains how you can restore and maintain health through the wise use of nutrients.

Part One of this easy-to-use guide discusses the individual nutrients necessary for good health. Part Two offers personalized nutritional programs for people with a wide variety of health concerns. People without prior medical problems can look to Part Three for their supplementation plans. Whether you want to maintain good health or you are trying to overcome a medical condition, *What You Must Know About Vitamins, Minerals, Herbs & More* can help you make the best choices for the well-being of you and your family.

*$15.95 US • 448 pages • 6 x 9-inch quality paperback • ISBN 978-0-7570-0233-5*

# JUICE ALIVE
## SECOND EDITION
### The Ultimate Guide to Juicing Remedies

Steven Bailey, ND,
and Larry Trivieri, Jr.

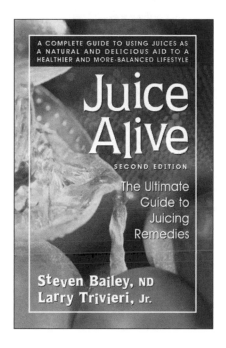

The juice of fresh fruits and vegetables provides a veritable powerhouse of antioxidants, vitamins, minerals, and enzymes. The trick is knowing which juices can best serve your individual needs. In this fascinating and easy-to-use guide, health experts Dr. Steven Bailey and Larry Trivieri, Jr. tell you everything you need to know to maximize the health benefits and tastes of juice.

The book begins with a unique look at the long history of juicing. It then examines the many components that make fresh juice truly good for you—good for weight loss, for renewed energy, and so much more. Next, it offers practical advice about the various types of juices available, as well as buying and storing tips for fruits, veggies, and herbs. The second half of the book begins with an important chart that matches up common ailments with the most appropriate juices, followed by over 100 delicious juice recipes. Also included is a juice cleansing regime and beauty aid program.

If you've never juiced before, let *Juice Alive* introduce you to a world bursting with the exciting tastes and incomparable benefits of fresh juice.

*$14.95 US • 272 pages • 6 x 9-inch quality paperback • ISBN 978-0-7570-0266-3*

# THE DŌ-IN WAY
## Gentle Exercises to Liberate the Body, Mind, and Spirit
### Michio Kushi

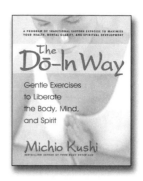

Dō-In is an ancient form of exercise that uses breathing techniques, posture, and self-massage and manipulation to stimulate body systems. Over the last 5,000 years, it has served as the origin of such well-known disciplines as shiatsu, acupuncture, moxibustion, yogic exercises, and meditation. *The Dō-In Way* is a comprehensive handbook to this system of movement designed to harmonize the body and cultivate physical health, mental serenity, and spirituality.

*$15.95 US • 224 pages • 7.5 x 9-inch quality paperback • ISBN 978-0-7570-0268-7*

# BIG YOGA
## A Simple Guide for Bigger Bodies
### Meera Patricia Kerr

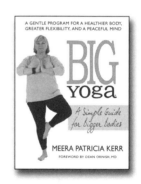

If you think yoga is only for skinny people, you need to think again. To expert Meera Patricia Kerr, yoga can and should be used by everyone—*especially* plus-size individuals. In her new book, *Big Yoga,* Meera shares the unique yoga program she developed for all those who think that yoga is not for them.

Part One of *Big Yoga* begins with a clear explanation of what yoga is, what benefits it offers, and how it can fit into anyone's life. Included is an important discussion of self-image. The book goes on to provide practical information regarding clothing, mats, and suitable environments, and to emphasize the need to begin with care. Part Two offers over forty different exercises specifically designed to work with bigger bodies. In each case, the author clearly explains the technique, details its advantages, and offers step-by-step instructions along with easy-to-follow photographs.

If you have thought that yoga is not for you, pick up *Big Yoga* and let Meera Patricia Kerr help you become more confident and relaxed than you may have ever thought possible.

*$17.95 US • 240 pages • 7.5 x 9-inch quality paperback • ISBN 978-0-7570-0215-1*

# WHAT YOU MUST KNOW ABOUT WOMEN'S HORMONES

## Your Guide to Natural Hormone Treatments for PMS, Menopause, Osteoporosis, PCOS, and More

Pamela Wartian Smith, MD, MPH

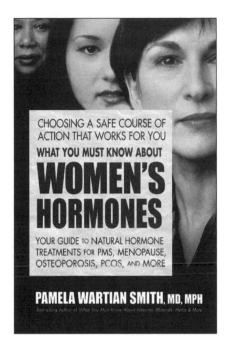

Hormonal imbalances can occur at any age and for a variety of reasons. While most related problems are generally associated with menopause, fluctuating hormonal levels can also cause a variety of other conditions, the effects of which can be debilitating. *What You Must Know About Women's Hormones* is a guide to the treatment of hormonal irregularities without the health risks associated with standard hormone replacement therapy.

This book is divided into three parts. Part One describes the body's own hormones, looking at their functions and the problems that can occur if they are not at optimal levels. Part Two focuses on the most common problems that arise from hormonal imbalances, such as PMS, hot flashes, postpartum depression, and endometriosis. Part Three details hormone replacement therapy, focusing on the difference between natural and synthetic treatments. Whether you are looking for help with menopausal symptoms or you simply want to enjoy vibrant health, *What You Must Know About Women's Hormones* can make a profound difference in the quality of your life.

*$17.95 US • 256 pages • 6 x 9-inch quality paperback • ISBN 978-0-7570-0307-3*

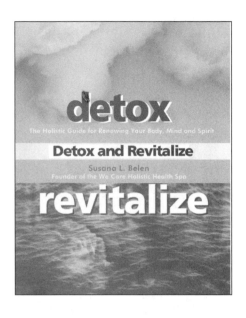

# Detox and Revitalize

## The Holistic Guide for Renewing Your Body, Mind, and Spirit

Susana Belen

Even if you try to follow a healthy diet and lifestyle, every day, toxins and waste materials accumulate in your cells, compromising your health. Fortunately, help is at hand. *Detox and Revitalize* is a complete guide to fasting, cleansing, and nutrition that will allow you to detox from daily air, food, and water pollutants; regain your natural vitality; and restore mental clarity and balance.

Part One of *Detox and Revitalize* explains the need for detoxification, and guides you in purifying your body from harmful substances. Part Two presents taste-tempting recipes for grains, cereals, and legumes; drinks and smoothies; salads; soups; main dishes; and even sweets that will increase your vitality. Helpful chapters on herbs and home remedies round out the book, providing all the information you need to ensure a healthier, more energetic future.

*$14.95 US • 160 pages • 8 x 10-inch quality paperback • ISBN 978-1-890612-46-7*